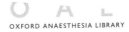

OXFORD ANAESTHESIA LIBRARY

Obstetric Anaesthesia for Developing Countries

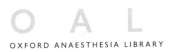

OXFORD ANAESTHESIA LIBRARY

Obstetric Anaesthesia for Developing Countries

Edited by

Dr Paul Clyburn

Consultant Anaesthetist, Department of Anaesthesia,
University Hospital of Wales, Cardiff, UK

Dr Rachel Collis

Consultant Anaesthetist, Department of Anaesthesia,
University Hospital of Wales, Cardiff, UK

Dr Sarah Harries

Consultant Anaesthetist, Department of Anaesthesia,
University Hospital of Wales, Cardiff, UK

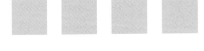

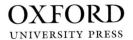

OXFORD
UNIVERSITY PRESS

OXFORD
UNIVERSITY PRESS

Great Clarendon Street, Oxford OX2 6DP

Oxford University Press is a department of the University of Oxford.
It furthers the University's objective of excellence in research, scholarship,
and education by publishing worldwide in

Oxford New York

Auckland Cape Town Dar es Salaam Hong Kong Karachi
Kuala Lumpur Madrid Melbourne Mexico City Nairobi
New Delhi Shanghai Taipei Toronto

With offices in

Argentina Austria Brazil Chile Czech Republic France Greece
Guatemala Hungary Italy Japan Poland Portugal Singapore
South Korea Switzerland Thailand Turkey Ukraine Vietnam

Oxford is a registered trade mark of Oxford University Press
in the UK and in certain other countries

Published in the United States
by Oxford University Press Inc., New York

British Library Cataloguing in Publication Data
Data available

Library of Congress Cataloging in Publication Data
Data available

Typeset by Newgen Imaging Systems (P) Ltd., Chennai, India
Printed in Great Britain
on acid-free paper by
Ashford Colour Press Ltd., Gosport, Hampshire

ISBN 978-0-19-957214-4

10 9 8 7 6 5 4 3 2 1

Whilst every effort has been made to ensure that the contents of this book are as
complete, accurate and-up-to-date as possible at the date of writing. Oxford
University Press is not able to give any guarantee or assurance that such is the case.
Readers are urged to take appropriately qualified medical advice in all cases. The
information in this book is intended to be useful to the general reader, but should
not be used as a means o self-diagnosis or for the prescription of medication.

Dedication

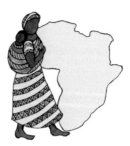

This pocketbook is dedicated to all mothers in Africa and other parts of the developing world who aspire to receive first world healthcare.

The Department of Anaesthetics in Cardiff is supporting education and training of healthcare professionals in the poorest countries of Africa through its registered charity:

Mothers of Africa
Registered No 1114509

Contents

Foreword

Obstetric Anaesthesia in Developing Countries is a collaborative effort by the Association of Anaesthetists of Great Britain and Ireland, the Obstetric Anaesthetists' Association and the World Federation of Societies of Anaesthesiologists.

It is well recognized that many millions of births take place each year where facilities for safe obstetric care are lacking. Anaesthesia is a key component of safe motherhood and yet is under-resourced as a specialty in many countries.

This book was conceived as a short text to describe how to provide practical safe anaesthesia for obstetric patients where resources are in short supply – a reality for many colleagues internationally. Although deficiencies make safe obstetric anaesthesia care difficult, there is much that the well trained and well informed anaesthesia provider can achieve, by using available resources in a timely and effective way.

This text describes a practical approach to setting up an anaesthesia service, administering both regional and general anaesthesia and managing complicated pregnancy and delivery, including neonatal resuscitation. It is hoped that the practical advice provided will prove helpful for colleagues striving to give their best care under all conditions.

Significant funding from the AAGBI, OAA and the WFSA means that thousands of these books will be made freely available to anaesthetists in developing countries. The advice in the book will be useful at all levels, not only for medical and non-medical anaesthesia providers, but also for obstetricians and midwives and all others in the obstetric team.

Dr Angela Enright
President – WFSA

Preface

This book was conceived to guide and inform all anaesthetists (regardless of background) who work in developing countries to safely manage pregnant mothers. The resources available to anaesthetists in developing countries are very variable and often limited, particularly in rural settings. This book, therefore, mainly emphasizes care that is possible regardless of resources and equipment. It does not simply concentrate on the process of giving a general or regional anaesthetic to a pregnant woman, but also on the physiological changes of pregnancy, assessment of the mother, management of pain relief during labour, and post delivery care. There are also sections on managing the sick and complicated pregnant woman. It is expected that although resources are often very limited, they are likely to steadily improve and we have therefore included techniques and facilities that, although may not be available at present, are something that can be aspired to in the future.

Obstetric anaesthesia requires close teamwork with other healthcare workers involved with the care of the mother and safe delivery of the baby. This book is also useful for obstetricians and midwifes who work in low resource situations.

Although the editors and principal authors are mostly UK based obstetric anaesthetists, most have experience of working in developing countries.

We are grateful to the Association of Anaesthetists of Great Britain and Ireland, the Obstetric Anaesthesia Association and the World Federation of Societies of Anaesthesiologists for their generous grants which should ensure that this book is distributed freely to anaesthesia providers working in resource poor countries.

With increasing availability of the internet, albeit intermittently in many places, the following link may be helpful to anaesthetists working in disadvantaged areas, providing access to WFSA educational resources such as Anaesthesia Update and Tutorial of the Week.

http://anaesthesiologists.org/en/education/wfsa-education-resources.html

In addition, the Association of Anaesthetists of GB and Ireland are developing resources to complement this book (http://www.aagbi.org) and the Obstetric Anaesthetists' Association have useful information on obstetric anaesthesia in different countries, including translations of patient information sheets (access through international tab at http://www.oaa-anaes.ac.uk).

Paul Clyburn
Rachel Collis
Sarah Harries

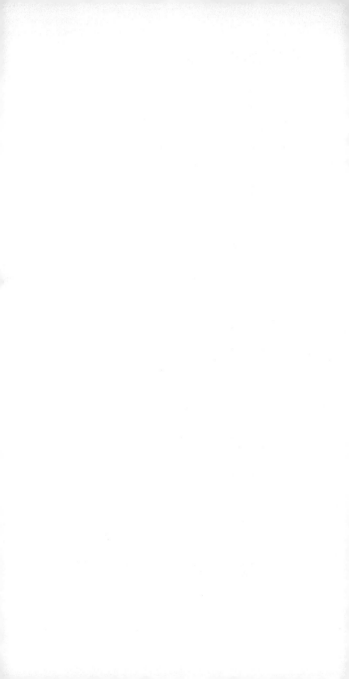

Symbols and abbreviations

AAGBI	Association of Anaesthetists of Great Britain and Ireland
ABC	Airway, Breathing, Circulation
ACE	angiotensin converting enzyme
ACT	artemisinin combination therapy
AF	atrial fibrillation
AFE	amniotic fluid embolism
ALP	alkaline phospatase
ALS	advanced life support
ALT	alanine transaminase
AP	anaesthetic practitioner
APTT	activated partial thromboplastin time
ARF	acute renal failure
ART	antiretroviral therapy
AST	aspartate transaminase
AVPU	Alert, responds to Voice, responds to Pain, Unconscious
BP	blood pressure
CEMACH	UK Report into Confidential Enquiries into Maternal and Child Health
CO	cardiac output
CRF	chronic renal failure
CRP	c-reactive protein
CS	caesarean section
CSE	combined spinal epidural
CSF	cerebrospinal fluid
CTG	cardiotocography
CTPA	computed tomographic pulmonary angiography
CVP	central venous pressure
DIC	disseminated intravascular coagulation
DVT	deep vein thrombosis
ECG	electrocardiogram

ECV	external cephalic version
FFP	fresh frozen plasma
FRC	functional residual capacity
GA	general anaesthesia
GFR	glomerular filtration rate
HELLP	Haemolytic anaemia, Elevated Liver enzymes and Low Platelets
HAART	highly active ART
HIV	Human Immunodeficiency Virus
HOCM	hypertrophic obstructive cardiomyopathy
IM	intramuscularly
ITN	insecticide treated mosquito nets
IV	intravenously
IVC	inferior vena cava
LA	local anaesthetic
LDH	lactate dehydrogenase
LEHPZ	lower oesophageal high-pressure zone
LMA	laryngeal mask airway
LMWH	Low molecular weight heparin
MAC	minimal alveolar concentration
MS	mitral stenosis
NCCEDM	National Committee on Confidential Enquiries into Maternal Deaths
NIBP	non-invasive blood pressure
NSAID	non steroidal anti inflammatory drugs
NVP	nevirapine
PCA	patient controlled analgesia
PCEA	patient controlled epidural analgesia
PCIA	patient controlled intravenous analgesia
PDPH	postdural puncture headache
PE	pulmonary embolus
PET	pre-eclampsia
PPCM	Peripartum Cardiomyopathy
PPH	postpartum haemorrhage
PPTp	intermittent preventive treatment during pregnancy
PTSD	post-traumatic stress disorder

SP	sulfadoxine-pyrimethamine
SVR	systemic vascular resistance
TAP	transversus abdominis plane
TENS	transcutaneous electrical nerve stimulation
TMJ	temporomandibular joint
UFH	unfractionated heparin
UTI	urinary tract infections
VBAC	vaginal delivery after CS
VF	ventricular fibrillation
V/Q	ventilation/perfusion
VT	ventricular tachycardia
VTE	venous thrombo-embolism
VQ	ventilation perfusion
WFSA	World Federation of Societies of Anaesthesiologists
WHO	World Health Organization
ZDV	zidovudine

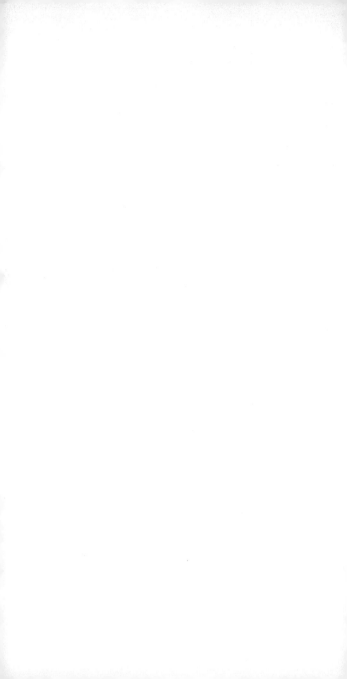

Contributors

Rafal Baraz
Department of Anaesthesia,
University Hospital of Wales,
Cardiff, UK

Sue Catling
Department of Anaesthetics,
Singleton Hospital, Sketty,
Swansea, UK

Paul Clyburn
Department of Anaesthesia,
University Hospital of Wales,
Cardiff, UK

Rachel Collis
Department of Anaesthesia,
University Hospital of Wales,
Cardiff, UK

Martin Garry
Department of Anaesthetics,
Singleton Hospital, Sketty,
Swansea, UK

Zipporah Gathuya
Gertrude's Children's Hospital,
Nairobi, Kenya

Sarah Harries
Department of Anaesthesia,
University Hospital of Wales,
Cardiff, UK

Saira Hussain
Department of Anaesthesia,
University Hospital of Wales,
Cardiff, UK

Eleanor Lewis
Department of Anaesthetics,
Singleton Hospital, Sketty,
Swansea, UK

Stephen Morris
Departments of Anaesthetics,
University Hospital Llandough,
Llandough, UK

Dermot Nicolson
Department of Anaesthesia,
University Hospital of Wales,
Cardiff, UK

Raman Sivasankar
Department of Anaesthesia,
Dunedin Hospital,
Dunedin, New Zealand

Isabeau Walker
Dept of Anaesthetics,
Great Ormond Hospital
for Children,
London, UK

Eugène Zoumenou
CNHU and HOMEL Hospitals,
Cotonou, Benin

Chapter 1

Setting up a maternity anaesthetic service

Martin Garry, Sarah Harries,
Rachel Collis

> **Key points**
> - Maternal mortality remains very high in many resource poor countries
> - A well managed obstetric anaesthetic service can help to reduce maternal mortality
> - Good standards of education of healthcare workers, basic resources and teamwork within hospitals are required
> - Audit and risk management can identify deficiencies, leading to changes which improve patient outcome.

1.1 Introduction

Maternal morbidity and mortality related to childbirth remain a huge challenge in many areas of the developing world, with estimated figures in some areas of Western Africa exceeding 1,000 maternal deaths per 100,000 live births. The successful prevention of further maternal deaths requires a commitment from all healthcare providers to deliver a high quality obstetric, midwifery and anaesthetic service within available resources.

Any successful healthcare service is dependent on the following key factors: a stable infrastructure, skilled personnel, a reliable stream of essential drugs and supplies, well-maintained equipment and a shared common goal to aspire to provide the best possible care to all mothers at all times.

When establishing or restructuring any maternity service, the anaesthetist and/or the anaesthetic practitioner (AP) plays a key role in ensuring the service provides safe general and regional anaesthesia for operative delivery, provides appropriate pain relief for women in labour and during the postnatal period, institutes a process for prompt recognition and resuscitation of a sick mother and provides continuing training, supervision and review of practice to encourage the service to develop.

1.2 Minimal standards for safe anaesthesia

International standards for the safe practice of anaesthesia have been defined and were adopted by the World Federation of Societies of Anaesthesiologists (WFSA) in 1992, and updated in 2008.

In addition to the WFSA minimum standards, the Association of Anaesthetists of Great Britain and Ireland (AAGBI) has published more comprehensive recommendations for standards of monitoring during anaesthesia and recovery (Table 1.1 and 1.2).

Table 1.1 Minimum requirements for safe anaesthesia	
General Anaesthesia	Oxygen supply
	Face masks
	Laryngoscope
	Tracheal tubes
	Suction apparatus
	Pulse oximeter
	Tilting table
	Intravenous cannulae and fluids
Spinal Anaesthesia	General anaesthesia requirements plus:
	Local anaesthetic +/– opioid drugs
	Sterile spinal needles
	Sterile syringes
	Disinfectant to clean skin
	Sterile gloves
	Blood pressure monitor
	Vasopressor drugs e.g. ephedrine, adrenaline
In addition for obstetric anaesthesia	GA and spinal anaesthesia requirements as above plus:
	Access to blood for transfusion
	Oxytocin or ergometrine
	Hydralazine or labetalol
	Magnesium sulphate

Table 1.2 AAGBI recommendations for standards of monitoring

Role of Anaesthetist/ Anaesthetic Practitioner (AP)	The continuous presence of an anaesthetist or an appropriately trained AP is mandatory throughout surgery under GA or a regional anaesthetic technique
Anaesthetic equipment	It is the responsibility of the anaesthetist or AP to check all equipment before use. **Essential monitoring equipment:** Oxygen analyzer with an audible alarm End-tidal capnography Vapour analyzer during volatile agent use All equipment should have audible alarms set with appropriate limits, including the ventilator alarms Provision, maintenance, calibration and renewal of equipment are the responsibility of the institution
Patient monitoring	Clinical observations during anaesthesia include: colour, pupil size, response to surgical stimulus, movement of the chest wall and reservoir bag, palpation of pulse, auscultation of breath sounds, measurement of urine output and blood loss **Essential intra-operative monitoring:** Pulse oximeter Non-invasive blood pressure monitoring Electrocardiograph Airway gases: oxygen, carbon dioxide, vapour Airway pressure Access to a peripheral nerve stimulator
Postoperative care	A high standard of monitoring should be continued during patient transfer and in the recovery room, until the patient is fully recovered from surgery Early warning score observation charts are useful in detecting small changes in pulse and BP, indicative of continuing bleeding

In addition to the above, there must be a clean theatre environment with sterile surgical equipment, a tilting operating table and good lighting. There should also be basic haematology laboratory services where blood can be x-matched and haemoglobin estimated, facility to warm fluids, and a reliable oxygen source.

In the postoperative period, the patient requires a post anaesthetic care area with monitors and oxygen so that the patient can be observed before safe discharge to ward.

1.3 **Role of the anaesthetist or anaesthetic practitioner**

The anaesthetist or anaesthetic practitioner (AP) is a key member of the maternity team, which also consists of the obstetrician and midwife. Each healthcare professional brings different skills to the team, which are necessary to provide a safe maternity service. Good communication, teamwork and professionalism are important to ensure that the best possible care and outcomes are achieved.

1.4 **Training of anaesthetic practitioners**

The training programme for APs varies between countries; however, it is usual for APs to complete a 3-year basic nursing course followed by a 2 year dedicated anaesthetic course prior to accreditation.

Core competencies required before working in maternity services are:

- Relevant technical skills i.e. intravenous access, advanced airway management, insertion of spinal +/− epidural techniques
- Knowledge of the physiology of pregnancy and how it differs from a non-pregnant female
- Awareness of common obstetric and anaesthetic emergencies and how to deal with them
- Confidence in the management of any adverse events or complications of anaesthesia
- Recognition and treatment of the seriously ill pregnant woman
- Proficiency in resuscitation of the mother and fetus.

1.5 **Developing an obstetric anaesthetic service**

1.5.1 **Teamwork**
The core to a successful obstetric anaesthetic service is that all members work successfully as a team. There should be regular joint review of patients by the anaesthetist, obstetrician and midwives. The views of all team members are important. If emergencies arise, clear communication between team members will improve patient safety and outcome for mother and baby.

1.5.2 **Protocols and guidelines**
When setting up an anaesthetic service, clinical guidelines can improve patient safety. There needs to be a consensus amongst clinical staff as to how procedures and emergencies are managed; this is then expressed as written guidelines which when followed ensure

consistent clinical practice. The main advantage of following written guidelines is that the anaesthetic service will run in a 'predictable' way, and can be understood by other members of the delivery ward team. Guidelines that cross specialities, especially those relating to the management of obstetric heamorrhage, hypertension and pre-eclampsia, should be written with the input and agreement of ALL team members (anaesthetic staff, obstetricians and midwives), and adhered to during patient treatment.

When the labour ward is quiet, the management of common emergencies should be regularly practiced as 'cold' simulation drills with someone pretending to be the patient, so that all staff become familiar with their role in successfully managing the emergency, e.g. major obstetric haemorrhage, cord prolapsed, shoulder dystocia, maternal collapse. Following the drill, an open discussion by the team of what went well and what could be done better can improve future performance of the real emergency.

1.5.3 **Audit**

'Audit is a quality improvement process that seeks to improve patient care and outcomes through systematic review of care against explicit criteria and the implementation of change' (NICE/CHI 2002). Through audit, patient care and safety is enhanced. When setting up an anaesthetic service, it is important to know the quantity of work that is being undertaken and also whether there are shortcomings that can be addressed.

1.5.3.1 *The audit cycle*

The audit cycle is a description of how audit ought to work in clinical practice, with continual assessment and feedback. You should:

- Set a standard
- Measure performance against that standard
- Diagnose the problem if the standard is not met, which will broadly fall into four categories of deficiency: knowledge, skills, attitude, organization
- Implement change
- Complete the cycle by remeasurement of performance.

The audit cycle is frequently broken. The measure of performance against a standard is easily determined, but analyzing the reasons behind a poor performance is complex and is often caused by many factors. Implementing change can be challenging and a return to the remeasure of performance at the end of the audit cycle may demon-strate how difficult it is to bring change into clinical practice.

1.5.3.2 Data collection

- **Quantitative data:** provides information on activity within a service and is important to establish adequate staffing levels and denominator numbers for qualitative audit
- **Qualitative data:** provides information on the quality of a service and the incidence of side effects.

1.6 Critical incident reporting and risk management

Even in the best circumstances, medical incidents occur with a poor or sub-optimal outcome for the mother or baby. For the service to improve and the number of incidents to fall, there has to be an open and frank discussion as to where the problems may have occurred. A well managed hospital or department will usually have a reporting system where, after a written report of the incident, senior team members review the case and make recommendations for change. If this does not exist, it is relatively easy to implement even in a low resource setting and can dramatically improve patient safety and care. Without a reporting system, it is very difficult to bring about improvements, particularly in dealing with recurring problems.

It is easy to blame an individual for an incident but usually the underlying cause is more complex. Although the incident may appear to have been caused by an individual, it is often the lack of education or equipment that is the underlying problem which needs addressing. For clinical incident reporting and risk management to be most effective, the group that analyse the reports and make recommendations should be from the anaesthetic team, obstetric team and midwives. Once a system has been set up which is NOT felt to be coercive, hospital staff will report freely, improvements in hospital care can be instituted and focused on improving patient safety and patient outcome.

1.7 WHO Surgical Safety Checklist

The World Health Organization has launched a second global patient safety challenge, 'Safe Surgery Saves Lives', to reduce the number of surgical deaths across the world. A core set of safety checks have been identified in the form of a WHO Surgical Safety Checklist for use in any operating theatre environment. This checklist has been widely adopted internationally and is available to download from www.who.int/patientsafety.

Chapter 2

Maternal physiology and pathophysiology

Dermot Nicolson, Rachel Collis

> **Key points**
> - Major physiological changes occur during pregnancy
> - These changes are brought about by hormonal factors and mechanical factors from the enlarging uterus
> - An understanding of these physiological changes is vital: they have implications for the safe care of the pregnant patient and conduct of anaesthesia
> - Knowledge of the physiological changes allows us to anticipate the effect that pregnancy will have on co-morbid medical conditions.

2.1 Cardiovascular system

2.1.1 Blood volume

The most striking maternal physiological alteration occurring during pregnancy is the increase in blood volume, which progresses throughout pregnancy. The average increase in blood volume at term is 45–50%. This is brought about by a 45% increase in plasma volume and a 20% increase in red blood cell volume. The disproportionate increase in plasma volume over red blood cells causes the physiological anaemia of pregnancy, where the average haemoglobin concentration falls by 2 g/dl. The increase in blood volume is needed to provide extra blood flow to the uterus, kidneys and to supply the extra metabolic needs of the fetus.

2.1.2 Haemodynamic changes in pregnancy

During pregnancy, there is an increase in the heart rate and stroke volume (the amount of blood pumped by the heart with each heart beat) producing a raised cardiac output (CO). The blood pressure does not increase despite the increase in cardiac output because there is a progressive fall in systemic vascular resistance (SVR). This fall in peripheral resistance results in a maximal decrease in mean arterial pressure by the end of the first trimester. The diastolic blood pressure (BP) falls between 5 and 15 mmHg, before rising to non-pregnant levels by term, while systolic BP remains unchanged throughout pregnancy. The heart rate increases from ~72 to 85 beats/minute and stroke volume increases by up to 30%. This, together with the reduction in SVR, increases the CO to a maximum of 50% above non-pregnant levels by 24 weeks gestation. The increased blood flow is distributed mainly to the uterus and kidneys. Uterine blood flow increases from 50 ml/minute at 10 weeks gestation to 850 ml/minute at term and renal blood flow increases by 80%.

2.1.3 Haemodynamic changes during labour

CO increases further during labour. Between uterine contractions, the CO increases from pre-labour values by 10–25% during the first stage of labour, and 40% during the second stage of labour. CO and SVR increase by a further 15–25% during contractions, and this increase can be reduced by effective epidural analgesia. A progressive rise in sympathetic nervous system activity, which peaks at the time of delivery, increases myocardial contractility, SVR, and venous return. An auto-transfusion of 500 ml blood, from the placenta into the circulation, occurs during the third stage.

2.1.4 Haemodynamic changes during the puerperium

There is a state of relative hypervolaemia and an increase in venous return following vaginal delivery with a sustained increase in cardiac output and central venous pressure. Mothers with significant cardiac disease are at increased risk during this period.

2.1.5 Haematological changes

The disproportionate increase in plasma volume over red cell volume in pregnancy causes a physiological anaemia, with a 15% drop in haemoglobin concentration and a decrease in blood viscosity. There is an increased demand for iron due to the increase in red cell volume and fetal requirements, and if iron stores are low, iron deficiency anaemia occurs. The platelets tend to remain normal but the white cell count increases during labour. Plasma protein concentration falls by 15% due to the increase in plasma volume, predisposing to the oedema seen in pregnancy and altering the pharmacokinetics of protein bound drugs. There is a relative hypercoagulable state during pregnancy in anticipation of haemorrhage at childbirth. This is brought about by an increase in clotting factors (V, VIII and X) and a decrease in fibrinolytic and protein C activity. Due to this hypercoagulable state, there is an increased risk of thromboembolic disease in pregnancy.

Aorto-caval compression

Aorto-caval compression occurs when the pregnant woman lies supine or semi-supine and the gravid uterus compresses the inferior vena cava (IVC) and aorta. This causes a decrease in venous return to the heart and a fall in CO and blood pressure, which can compromise the mother or fetus. The reduction in venous return is partly compensated for by increased distal venous pressure pushing blood through the compressed IVC, and by collateral venous pathways. Maternal symptoms and signs range from asymptomatic or mild hypotension, to total cardiovascular collapse. During regional anaesthesia, symptoms of dizziness, feeling faint and nausea often indicate a decrease in blood pressure. The severity of aorto-caval compression may depend on:

- The effectiveness of collateral venous systems
- Gestation, with maximal effect seen at 36–38 weeks
- Large uterine size associated with multiple pregnancies or polyhydramnios
- The presence of a sympathetic block from anaesthesia.

A woman who is not anesthetized may be able to compensate for a drop in BP by increasing her SVR. However, in anaesthetized patients, these compensatory mechanisms are reduced or abolished resulting in a greater fall in BP when aorto-caval compression occurs. Even in the absence of maternal symptoms, placental blood supply may be compromised in the supine position, and after the 20th week of gestation, a left lateral tilt should ALWAYS be maintained to prevent aorto-caval compression. This tilt can be achieved by placing a wedge under the mother's hip, tilting the operating table by 15 degrees to the left, or placing the mother in the full lateral position.

2.2 Respiratory system

Hormonal and mechanical factors during pregnancy cause major physiological and anatomical changes in the respiratory system.

2.2.1 Anatomical changes

Hormonal changes result in capillary engorgement and swelling of the mucosa of the nose, oropharynx, larynx and trachea. This may be exacerbated by pre-eclampsia or fluid overload. As a result, smaller tracheal tubes might be required for intubation and bleeding may be precipitated by the use of nasal tubes, nasogastric tubes or oral/nasal airways. The enlarging uterus displaces the diaphragm upwards, but the volume of the thoracic cage remains the same due to an increase in both the antero-posterior and transverse chest diameters.

2.2.2 Ventilatory changes

There is a progressive increase in oxygen consumption in pregnancy caused by the increased metabolic needs of the mother and fetus. Oxygen consumption increases by 20–30% at term. During labour, it is increased by 60% as a result of the increased cardiac and respiratory workload. This is compensated for by the effect of progesterone stimulating respiration and enhancing the response of the respiratory centre to carbon dioxide (CO_2). There is a 45–50% increase in minute ventilation caused by an increase in tidal volume, and to a lesser extent respiratory rate. The tidal volume increases from ~500ml to 700ml. During labour, ventilation may be further accentuated in response to pain or anxiety. Ventilation in pregnancy is greater than the body's demand for oxygen and CO_2 production, which causes CO_2 to be washed out of the lungs creating a respiratory alkalosis with $PaCO_2$ falling from 5 to 4 kPa. This mild alkalaemia improves oxygen release to the fetus. Although the minute ventilation increases during pregnancy and labour, this increase is trivial in comparison to the increases which occur during exercise i.e. a 10-fold increase. This considerable respiratory reserve explains why respiratory failure due to chronic respiratory disease is uncommon in pregnancy.

2.2.3 Volume changes

The enlarging uterus causes a 4 cm elevation of the diaphragm, but the total lung capacity only decreases by 5% because the lower ribs flare out, increasing the transverse and antero-posterior diameters of the chest. Despite the upward displacement of the diaphragm, it moves with greater excursion in the pregnant woman. The functional residual capacity (FRC), which is the volume of air remaining in the lung at the end of a normal breath, decreases by 20% as pregnancy progresses due to the increased intra-abdominal pressure and upward displacement of the diaphragm. Closing capacity (lung volume at which airway closure occurs) can encroach on the FRC, but remains less than the FRC while the patient is in the upright position. During the second half of pregnancy, closing capacity is greater than FRC in 50% of pregnant woman when she lies down. This causes airway closure in the dependant part of the lung, an increase in ventilation/perfusion (V/Q) mismatch and predisposes to hypoxia.

> ## Clinical implications of respiratory changes
>
> The combination of increased oxygen consumption and decreased FRC means that a pregnant mother who is rendered apnoeic at term, will desaturate much more quickly than her non-pregnant counterpart. This fall in blood oxygen saturation will be worse in women with twin or triplet pregnancies and the morbidly obese patient. Good preoxygenation is therefore essential in all pregnant women before general anaesthesia. The increase in minute ventilation and decrease in FRC hastens inhalation induction or changes in depth of anaesthesia when breathing spontaneously. Airway management is more challenging in pregnancy. Laryngoscopy may be difficult due to weight gain and breast engorgement. Instrumentation of the airway can cause profuse bleeding from the nose or oropharynx, especially when there is fluid overload or oedema associated with pre-eclampsia, making intubation even more difficult.

2.2.4 Respiratory disease

An increasing number of women with respiratory disease are becoming pregnant: the incidence of asthma is increasing and pulmonary tuberculosis remains a problem in developing countries. Respiratory disease may be exacerbated by the increased respiratory demands of pregnancy and labour, although asthma often improves during pregnancy. Women with severe respiratory disease should be seen early in pregnancy and have pulmonary function tests. Women with mild respiratory disease can be treated as normal. In patients with moderate to severe disease, epidural analgesia can help to reduce the stress of labour. If available, pulse oximetry monitoring is useful for labour in women with respiratory disease. For caesarean section, spinal anaesthesia avoids the depressant effects of general anaesthetic drugs but care must be taken to avoid a high spinal block.

2.3 Gastrointestinal system

2.3.1 Gastric function

Anatomical changes and hormonal effects on smooth muscle tone promote gastric contents to reflux into the oesophagus during pregnancy. The enlarging uterus increases gastric reflux in two ways. Firstly, the stomach is shifted upwards, and the lower intra-abdominal segment of the oesophagus is displaced up into the thorax, which reduces the effectiveness of the lower oesophageal sphincter, also known as the lower oesophageal high-pressure zone (LEHPZ). Secondly, the uterus compresses the intra-abdominal contents and increases intra-gastric pressure. Progesterone is a smooth muscle relaxant, and it also reduces the tone of the LEHPZ. Delayed gastric emptying will increase the residual volume in the stomach. There is no delay in gastric emptying during pregnancy and early labour, but some delay occurs just before delivery. However, gastric emptying is considerably slowed down by the use of opiate pain relief during labour. The risk of regurgitation decreases post delivery and should be normal 48 hours postpartum.

Clinical implications

Pulmonary aspiration of gastric contents can occur after vomiting or passive regurgitation, resulting in significant morbidity and mortality. All pregnant women should be considered to have a full stomach, with increased risk of aspiration from the end of the first trimester. During general anaesthesia, the airway needs to be protected with a cuffed tracheal tube. A rapid sequence induction should be performed with pre-oxygenation, cricoid pressure, and avoiding positive pressure ventilation until the airway is secured with a tracheal tube. The use of regional anaesthesia for caesarean section avoids the risks of aspiration associated with general anaesthesia.

2.3.2 Hepatic function

Changes in hepatic synthetic function and metabolism occur during pregnancy. Plasma concentrations of fibrinogen, ceruloplasmin, transferin, and binding proteins such as thyroid-binding globulin increase. Total body albumin also increases, but the serum albumin levels fall by 20% because of the increased blood volume. Many liver enzymes are increased to the upper limits of their normal ranges including AST, ALT and LDH. A 400% increase in ALP may occur due to placental production of the enzyme. Certain signs of liver disease such as telengiectasia and palmer erythema are common signs in normal pregnancy and resolve postpartum

2.4 Renal system

2.4.1 Renal function

Renal blood flow increases by 80% during pregnancy, causing the kidney to swell and increase in size, appearing 1cm longer on ultrasound. The renal pelvis and ureters dilate under the influence of progesterone, which is enhanced by the enlarging uterus producing partial obstruction of the ureters. There is a large increase in glomerular filtration rate (GFR) by the end of the first trimester leading to increased clearance of urea and creatinine. During pregnancy, urea and creatinine levels are 40% lower than non-pregnant values. The normal values therefore need to be adjusted as values within the normal range for the non-pregnant state may indicate significant renal function impairment during pregnancy. Proteinuria increases during pregnancy, but levels above 0.3 g in 24 hours should be considered abnormal

2.4.2 Renal disease

Pregnant women are at increased risk of urinary tract infections (UTI) which if untreated will develop into acute pyelonephritis in ~20% of cases. Symptoms of acute pyelonephritis include: fever, chills, flank pain and other symptoms of lower UTI. The causative organisms are usually E. coli, Klebsiella, and Proteus. Useful antibiotics for the treatment of UTI's include nitrofurantoin (not in first trimester), trimethoprim, ampicillin and cephalosporins. Pregnancy may predispose to the formation of renal stones in some susceptible women, which can be extremely painful, difficult to manage and may lead to acute renal failure (ARF).

The classification and some causes of ARF in pregnancy are:

- **Pre-renal:** hypovolaemia caused by haemorrhage, hyperemesis gravidarum and dehydration, and low cardiac output states
- **Renal:** Pre-eclampsia, eclampsia, HELLP syndrome, septic abortion, amniotic fluid embolus, pyelonephritis, acute tubular necrosis, and glomerulonephritis
- **Post-renal:** Renal stones, ureteral obstruction.

ARF is characterized by a rapid rise in serum creatinine (>73 mmol/L) and urea levels (>4.3 mmol/L), and urine output may fall to <400mL/day. ARF is not common in pregnancy and usually reflects severe underlying disease that requires urgent diagnosis and treatment. In women with chronic renal failure (CRF), the chances of becoming pregnant decrease with declining renal function and pregnancy is rare if the kidneys are functioning at less than 50% efficiency. Pregnant women with CRF are at high risk of developing pre-eclampsia and IUGR, with a high perinatal mortality. The increase in GFR during pregnancy will cause further damage to kidneys which are already impaired, and the woman's own condition is likely to deteriorate. Chronic renal impairment leads to activation of the renin-angiotensin system resulting in salt and water retention, and hypertension. The outcome of pregnancy depends on the degree of renal impairment, the blood pressure and episodes of infection. Termination of pregnancy or early induction of labour may be offered if the mother's condition is deteriorating. Women with CRF prior to pregnancy may never recover pre-pregnancy renal function if renal function deteriorates.

2.5 **Endocrine system**

The pituitary gland increases in size and prolactin, the hormone responsible for milk production, increases. Corticotrophin and cortisol levels increase, and together with placental lactogen, lead to insulin resistance which favours hyperglycaemia and the development of gestational diabetes. During pregnancy, thyroxine-binding globulin, thyroxine (T4) and tri-iodothyronine (T3) concentrations increase but the pregnant woman should remain euthyroid, as the levels of free T3 and T4 remain unchanged. There is an increased renal clearance of iodine and a relative state of iodine deficiency may develop, leading to enlargement of the thyroid gland.

2.6 **Central nervous system**

During pregnancy the changes in central nervous system physiology include changes in pain threshold, susceptibility to general and local anaesthetics (LA), and alterations in mood and cognitive function. The pharmacological response to general and LA are brought about by increased concentrations of progesterone and endogenous opioids (β-endorphins). The minimal alveolar concentration (MAC) for volatile anaesthetic agents are decreased and the amount of LA required to block nerve conduction is reduced. During pregnancy a given dose of intrathecal or epidural LA blocks more dermatomes than in non-pregnant patients. This may be due to increased susceptibility of nerve fibres to local anaesthetics, but the anatomical changes in the epidural space that occur during pregnancy also contribute. Engorgement of epidural veins caused by aorto-caval compression leads to a reduction in the volume available for the spread of LA within the vertebral canal. Therefore, an identical volume of LA will spread more extensively in the pregnant state.

Chapter 3

Maternal pharmacology

Dermot Nicolson, Rachel Collis

> ### Key points
> - Pregnancy results in changes in the pharmacokinetics and pharmacodynamics of drugs
> - The fetus may be affected by drugs administered to the mother
> - Drugs may pass from the mother to baby through breast milk
> - Knowledge of commonly used drugs is important for safe clinical practice.

3.1 Basic principles

Physiological, anatomical and hormonal changes in pregnancy alter the pharmacokinetics and pharmacodynamics of administered drugs.

3.1.1 Pharmacokinetics

3.1.1.1 Absorption

There is little change in the absorption of drugs during pregnancy. However, the increase in minute ventilation and decrease in FRC quickens the absorption of volatile anaesthetics, and vomiting associated with pregnancy can limit the absorption of orally administered drugs.

3.1.1.2 Distribution

The increase in body fluid and blood volume results in a greater volume of distribution and the increased cardiac output will redistribute drugs more quickly. The decrease in albumin and plasma proteins will increase the effect of protein bound drugs and changes in plasma pH, which can occur during labour from hyperventilation (alkalaemia) or exhaustion (acidaemia), may affect protein binding of drugs.

3.1.1.3 Metabolism

Plasma cholinesterase levels decrease during pregnancy prolonging the duration of action of suxamethonium. Drugs metabolized by the liver will be normal unless there is liver impairment as can occur in HELLP syndrome.

3.1.1.4 Elimination

Volatile anaesthetic agents are eliminated more rapidly due to the increased minute ventilation. The increased glomerular filtration rate seen in pregnancy results in a more rapid clearance of renally excreted drugs.

3.1.2 Pharmacodynamics

The minimal alveolar concentration of volatile anaesthetics is reduced and lower concentrations of local anaesthetic (LA) are required in pregnancy. The lower dose of epidural or spinal LA required in pregnancy is due to the effects of progesterone and a decrease in the epidural space volume caused by engorgement of the epidural veins.

3.1.3 Placental transfer of drugs

Almost all drugs administered to the mother will reach the fetus by crossing the placenta. Despite being a complex anatomical structure, the placenta behaves like a semi-permeable membrane with drugs crossing by diffusion. The factors affecting placental drug transfer are maternal drug concentration, drug molecular weight, degree of ionization, degree of protein binding and lipid solubility.

Most anaesthetic drugs are small and lipid soluble. They cross the placenta easily and their effects are only significant immediately post delivery. An exception to this, are the neuromuscular blocking drugs which are ionized and therefore not very lipid soluble. They do not cross the placenta when given in normal doses and have no effect on the fetus. Opiate analgesics cross the placenta and cause respiratory depression and reduced suckling ability in the new-born, which can be reversed by naloxone.

3.1.4 Drugs and breastfeeding

Medication should only be prescribed to breastfeeding mothers when necessary and the safest available drug should be chosen. Breastfeeding is the gold standard in infant nutrition and the risks of potential harm to the baby need to be balanced with the advantages of continued breastfeeding. Most drugs will enter breast milk but are usually present in insignificant amounts and will not pose a risk to the breastfed baby. Volatile and intravenous anaesthetic drugs are found in insignificant amounts in breast milk following general anaesthesia. An exception is etomidate, and breastfeeding should be withheld for 24 hours after its administration. The large, ionized and water insoluble neuromuscular blocking drugs are not excreted into breast milk. Paracetamol, non-steroidal anti-inflammatory (ibuprofen, diclofenac) and opioids (morphine, diamorphine, codeine, tramadol) are safe for postoperative pain relief in the breastfeeding mother.

3.2 **Intravenous induction agents**

3.2.1 **Thiopental**

Thiopental induces rapid, predictable anaesthesia, making it the easiest drug to use with suxamethonium and it remains the gold standard for a rapid sequence induction. At a dose of 4–6mg/kg there is reliable anaesthesia for 5–7 min, which allows the brain concentration of volatile anaesthetic agent to come up to a sleep dose at the start of anaesthesia. Rapid redistribution of thiopental in the maternal and fetal circulation allows the baby to be born with little sedation. However, at higher doses (8mg/kg) fetal depression will occur.

3.2.2 **Propofol**

Propofol is not considered as the first choice induction agent in obstetric anaesthesia because it lacks a clear induction endpoint, making it a difficult drug to use for a rapid sequence induction. The induction dose of propofol is 1–2mg/kg. Doses greater than 2.5mg/kg are associated with neonatal sedation. Propofol has a short duration of action due to redistribution and rapid wakening may be associated with an increased risk of maternal awareness.

3.2.3 **Ketamine**

Ketamine is not an ideal induction agent as it has a slow onset of action and the anaesthesia end-point is difficult to detect. However, it has been used for induction in haemodynamically compromised mothers as it does not cause the hypotension seen with thiopental and propofol. The induction dose is 1–2mg/kg. At 1mg/kg the neonate is born without sedation; however, a dose of 2mg/kg, which is a better induction dose, will result in neonatal depression. Other side effects of ketamine include hallucinations and delirium on waking.

3.2.4 **Etomidate**

Etomidate has been used to induce anaesthesia in haemodynamically compromised women as it does not cause hypotension. Anaesthesia can be induced at a dose of 0.3 mk/kg and the neonate will be born without sedation. It has many side effects including pain on injection, myoclonic rigidity and involuntary movements. It also inhibits adrenal cortisol production, which is associated with an adverse outcome in critically ill patients. Neonatal cortisol levels at 1 hour of age are also reduced, and this may be detrimental to an already compromised neonate.

3.3 **Inhalational agents**

Inhalational agents are used to maintain general anesthesia. The agents which are non-irritant to the airway may also be used for induction of anaesthesia. However, in obstetric anaesthesia, inhalational induction should be avoided because of the risk of aspiration. The potencies of volatile anaesthetics are described by their minimal alveolar concentration (MAC), which is the concentration that produces a lack of reflex movement in 50% of non-paralyzed patients when the skin is incised. To minimize the dose dependent uterine relaxation seen with volatiles, and help to prevent postpartum haemorrhage, they should be restricted to **0.5 MAC and used with nitrous oxide.** Volatile agents all cause dose and time dependent neonatal depression and induction to delivery time should be kept to less than 11 minutes.

3.3.1 **Halothane**

Halothane is a potent agent with a MAC of 0.75. It has a sweet odour and is non-irritant making it a good agent for inhalational induction of anaesthesia. It causes concentration dependent hypotension by depressing the myocardium and is commonly associated with arrhythmias. Like most volatile agents, it depresses the respiratory centre. Halothane undergoes hepatic metabolism (20%) and has been associated with severe hepatotoxicity with a high mortality. The hepatotoxicity is more likely after repeated exposure to halothane.

3.3.2 **Enflurane**

Enflurane has a MAC of 1.68. It is less cardio-depressant and arrhythmogenic than halothane. Enflurane causes more respiratory depression than the other agents. It undergoes less hepatic metabolism (2%) than halothane and is unlikely to cause hepatic toxicity. Enflurane may cause seizure like activity and should be avoided in epileptics.

3.3.3 **Isoflurane**

Isoflurane has a MAC of 1.17. It causes myocardial depression, but less so than enflurane or halothane, and dose related vasodilatation causes hypotension. A reflex tachycardia is seen in response to the drop in blood pressure. It depresses ventilation more than halothane but less so than enflurane and is irritant to the airway.

3.3.4 **Sevoflurane**

Sevoflurane has a low blood:gas solubility coefficient resulting in a rapid onset of action and rapid emergence from anaesthesia. It also has a pleasant odour making it a useful agent for induction of anaesthesia. It has a MAC of 1.8. Sevoflurane causes vasodilatation and causes hypotension with no change in heart rate. When used in a circle system with soda lime, a substance called Compound A is produced which is nephrotoxic in rats, but the concentrations produced are too small to have an effect on human renal function.

3.3.5 Ether

Although no longer used in many parts of the world, it remains a safe option in some low resource settings. It can be used as part of an open or draw-over anaesthetic technique, as it is sweet smelling, relatively non-irritant and does not cause respiratory depression around MAC concentration. It has a blood/gas solubility coefficient of 12 making it very slow in onset and waking from anaesthesia. MAC is 1.9 and care must be taken as it is flammable in air and oxygen at this concentration.

3.3.6 Nitrous oxide

Nitrous oxide is a weak anaesthetic agent that is insufficient to provide anaesthesia as a sole agent. It is a useful carrier gas used alongside the volatile agents and oxygen during general anaesthesia. Concentrations of >50% are associated with neonatal depression. Nitrous oxide 50% in oxygen is used initially with a volatile agent, and after delivery of the baby, it can be increased to 70% nitrous oxide and 30% oxygen. Nitrous oxide 70% in oxygen decreases the MAC of halothane to 0.29, enflurane to 0.6 and isoflurane to 0.5. Its main advantage is that it does not cause uterine relaxation and can be used to reduce the concentration of volatile agent required. Side effects include bone marrow suppression when used for prolonged periods, and nausea and vomiting. It causes an increase in the volume of gas filled spaces such as a pneumothorax or air emboulus, and if either of these conditions is suspected, the nitrous oxide should be turned off and replaced with 100% oxygen.

3.4 Muscle relaxants

3.4.1 Depolarizing muscle relaxant: suxamethonium

Suxamethonium produces muscle relaxation by depolarization of the post junctional membrane of the motor end-plate with characteristic fasciculations. When given in a dose of 1–1.5mg/kg there is maximal relaxation by 60 seconds. It is rapidly metabolized by plasma cholinesterase and normal muscle function returns within 5 minutes, unless the patient has low levels of this enzyme caused by a genetic deficiency or acquired through poisoning or slightly low levels due to pregnancy. If given in repeated doses or as an infusion it should be given with atropine to prevent bradycardia and the muscle paralysis can become prolonged. It MUST be kept refrigerated at all times as it is naturally hydrolyzed at room temperature and will become ineffective. It MUST NOT be used if the patient has a high potassium, extensive burns or major muscle paralysis. In normal doses placental transfer is minimal.

3.4.2 **Non-depolarizing muscle relaxants**

Act by competitive inhibition of the acetylcholine receptor on the motor end-plate. They are highly ionized and do not cross the placenta in normal doses. They are all renally excreted except atra-curium which under-goes spontaneous degradation. Atracurium is therefore the best drug if the patient has renal failure. Onset typically occurs 3–5 minutes after IV injection, depending on the dose, and lasts 20–60 minutes. These drugs should be reversed using neostig-mine 2.5–5mg with atropine or glycopyralate to prevent bradycardia. Neostigmine increases acetylcholine at the neuromuscular junction displacing the muscle relaxant. It is not possible to reverse these drugs until there is evidence of some return of neuromuscular func-tions which can be assessed with a peripheral nerve stimulator.

Atracurium: Requires refrigeration and in dose of 0.3–0.5mg/kg works in 2 minutes and lasts for 30 minutes. After suxamethonium the dose can be reduced by 50%. To maintain paralysis, additional doses of 25% of initial bolus can be given.

Vecuronium: Is stored as a powder and requires mixing in sterile water. Initial dose of 0.1mg/kg with repeat dose of 0.015mg/kg. Onset in this dose is 3 minutes and lasts for 20–30 minutes. Reduce the dose by 50% after suxamethonium.

Rocuronium: Requires refrigeration and in a dose of 0.6mg/kg has the most rapid on-set of action of 1.5–2 minutes and lasts for 45–60 minutes.

Pancuronium: Is slowest in onset making it the least suitable drug to facilitate a rapid sequence induction if suxamethonium is not available (see page 91). The dose is 0.1mg/kg with additional doses of 0.015mg/kg. It produces a release of noradrenaline and may cause a slight tachycardia with hypertension.

3.5 **Opioids**

Opioid analgesic drugs exert their effects by acting on opioid recep-tors and are used to treat severe pain. Side effects common to all opioids are dose dependent respiratory depression of mother and neonate, delayed gastric emptying, nausea and vomiting, sedation, euphoria, amnesia, and hypotension. The effects of opiates can be reversed with the antagonist naloxone.

3.5.1 **Pethidine**

Pethidine is a synthetic opioid analgesic drug widely used in the man-agement of labour pain. It is one-tenth as potent as morphine, with a duration of action between 2–4 hours. It has an active metabolite, norpethidine, which may cause hallucinations and convulsions. For obstetric analgesia, it is given as 100mg IM and repeated once (maximum 200mg). It has high lipid solubility and significant amounts cross the placenta. The babies of mothers who receive pethidine have been shown to be sleepier and slower to establish feeding. Pethidine is contraindicated in patients with pre-eclampsia or renal impairment.

3.5.2 Morphine

Morphine is a naturally occurring opioid and has low lipid solubility. It is bound to albumin in the circulation and readily crosses the placenta. Morphine is metabolized by the liver and one of the metabolites, morphine-6-glucuronide, has analgesic activity. The metabolites are excreted in the urine. Morphine can be administered orally, IM, IV, and intrathecally. The oral dose of morphine is 5–20mg 4 hourly and the intramuscular dose is 0.1-0.2mg/kg 4 hourly. The intravenous dose is 0.05–0.1mg/kg, but it should be titrated to effect. The dose in the epidural space is 4mg and should only be given once in 24hours and intrathecally 0.1–0.2mg once in 24 hours. Delayed respiratory depression may occur following epidural or intrathecal administration and should only be used by this route if the patient can receive regular respiratory rate monitoring for 24 hours after administration. The usual doses for maternal labour analgesia are 2–5mg IV or 5–10mg IM. The onset of analgesia is within 5 minutes after IV administration and within 20–40 minutes after IM administration.

3.5.3 Fentanyl

Fentanyl is a synthetic opioid with a rapid onset of action. It is very lipid soluble and highly bound to albumin. It is 100 times more potent than morphine. Fentanyl is used to augment the effect of local anaesthetic in spinal (10–25mcg) and epidural anaesthesia (2–5mcg/ml). Unlike morphine, it does not cause delayed respiratory depression as it has high lipid solubility and diffuses rapidly from the CSF into the spinal cord.

3.6 Local anaesthetics

Local anaesthetics (LA) produce temporary blockade of neural transmission by crossing the axon membrane, blocking the sodium channel, and preventing conduction of action potentials in the nerve. Only unionized LA can cross the axon cell membrane. The degree of ionization depends on the pK_a of the drug. LA's with a low pK_a are relatively more unionized and therefore have a fast onset of action. The duration of LA action depends on the degree of plasma protein binding. Extensive protein binding results in a long duration of action. The potency of LA is related to its lipid solubility.

3.6.1 **Lidocaine**

Lidocaine is the standard LA against which others are compared. It is presented as a 0.5–5% solution with or without added adrenaline. It has a pK_a of 7.9 resulting in a rapid onset of action. The duration of action is short (1 hour for 1% solution, increasing to 1.5–2 hours if adrenaline is added) due to its low protein binding of 65%. Maximum recommended doses are 3mg/kg without adrenaline and 7mg/kg with adrenaline.

3.6.2 **Bupivacaine**

Bupivacaine, with a pK_a of 8.1 has a slower onset of action compared with lidocaine, and a longer duration of action due to high protein binding (95%). Bupivacaine is presented as 0.25%, 0.5% and 0.75% solutions. The 0.75% solution should not be used in obstetrics because of the risk of toxicity. A hyperbaric 0.5% solution containing 8% glucose is available for spinal anaesthesia. Bupivacaine is more cardiotoxic than lidocaine and the maximum safe dose is 2mg/kg. Levobupivacaine, a newer and more expensive preparation which contains a single isomer of bupivacaine, has less toxicity.

3.6.3 **Ropivacaine**

Ropivacaine is presented as 0.2–1.0% solutions. It is chemically related to bupivacaine, but it is less lipid soluble and thus less potent. Onset and duration of action is similar to bupivacaine (pK_a 8.1 and 94% protein bound). It was believed that ropivacaine produced less motor block than bupivacaine when used epidurally, but this is now known to be due to its reduced potency, and at equipotent doses the incidence of motor block is similar. The maximum safe dose is 3.5mg/kg.

3.7 **Vasopressors**

Vasopressors cause vasoconstriction and are used to increase arterial blood pressure (BP). Historically, ephedrine was considered to be the vasopressor of choice in obstetric patients. This was based on animal research which showed that ephedrine maintained uterine blood flow, whereas, pure α_1 agonists such as phenylephrine reduced uterine blood flow. α_1 agonists have now been shown to be safe in pregnant women.

3.7.1 **Ephedrine**

Ephedrine is a direct α_1 and β receptor agonist and also acts indirectly by releasing noradrenaline (α_1 agonist) from nerve endings. It increases BP by augmenting CO through its actions on β-receptors and vasoconstriction through its α_1-receptor activity. The β effect increases CO by increasing heart rate and cardiac contractility, resulting in increased myocardial oxygen demand, which can be detrimental in patients with cardiac disease. Ephedrine has no or little effect on placental and uterine blood flow making it a useful drug in pregnant patients. It is an easy drug to use and can be given IV, IM or orally. It is commonly given as a 6mg IV bolus, repeated as required. Ephedrine has a slow onset of action and a long duration of action. With repeated administration, tachyphylaxis (a decrease in response to repeated doses) may occur as noradrenaline stores become depleted from nerve endings. Ephedrine has been associated with a small decrease in umbilical artery pH as a result of it crossing the placenta and stimulating fetal metabolism. This small drop in pH has not been shown to have a clinically significant effect on the neonate.

3.7.2 **Phenylephrine**

Phenylephrine is a direct α_1-receptor agonist causing vasoconstriction and a rise in BP. Human research has now shown that phenylephrine is a safe drug to use in pregnancy and there are no adverse fetal or neonatal effects when used in appropriate doses. It has a rapid onset and a short duration of action and can be administered by IV boluses of 12.5–50mcg, as required. Due to its short duration of action, it can also be administered as an infusion. A typical infusion would be 12.5mcg/ml infused at 80–100 ml/hr and titrated to effect. A reflex bradycardia is common with phenylephrine, which may need treatment with atropine or glycopyrronium, although it is uncommon for the heart rate to fall below 50bpm and rapidly reverses with cessation of use. Phenylephrine is supplied in a variety of concentrations (12.5mcg/ml, 250mcg/ml, 10mg/ml) and extreme care is needed when using it to ensure that the correct dose is given.

3.8 **Drugs for uterine contraction**

Uterotonic drugs play an important role following delivery and in the puerperium. They cause uterine contraction, aid expulsion of the placenta, and thus reduce postpartum haemorrhage (PPH) in patients with an atonic uterus. They may also be used to augment contractions during labour.

3.8.1 **Oxytocin**

Oxytocin analogue increases the force and frequency of uterine contractions. It is used to enhance contractions during labour and to control PPH. Following IM injection, the onset of action is 3–7 min, and lasts for 30–60 min. After IV injection, the myotonic effect appears within 1 min and has a short duration of action. It is usually given as a slow 5 IU bolus IV following caesarean delivery and can be continued as an infusion (30–50 IU in 500mL crystalloid over 4 hours). Side effects include hypotension, nausea and decreased urine output and water intoxication with hyponatraemia, due to an anti-diuretic effect.

3.7.2 **Ergomertrine**

Ergometrine is commonly given as an IM injection together with oxytocin in a combination called Syntometrine® (Ergometrine 500mcg and oxytocin 5 IU) at vaginal delivery. Ergometrine may also be given as a slow IV bolus. Following IM injection, uterine contractions start within 2–5 min and persist for more than 3 hours. Side effects include nausea and vomiting, headache, vasoconstriction, and hypertension. It is contraindicated in patients with hypertension, pre-eclampsia, heart disease, and hepatic or renal impairment.

3.7.3 **Carboprost (Hemabate®)**

Carboprost is a prostaglandin ($PGF_{2\alpha}$) and is only used to treat PPH when oxytocin and ergometrine have been ineffective at stopping the bleeding. It is given at a dose of 250mcg by deep IM injection or directly into the myometrium (dangerous if given IV). It can be administered at 90 minute intervals up to a maximum dose of 2mg, although a repeat dose can be given after 15 minutes if the bleeding is severe. With increasing doses, there is a risk of pulmonary oedema. Other side effect include bronchospasm (avoid in asthmatics), pyrexia, flushing, nausea and vomiting.

3.7.4 **Misoprostol**

Misoprostol, a prostaglandin analogue (PGE_1) and is the third or fourth choice drug for the treatment of uterine atony in the UK. It has, however, been shown to be effective as a first line drug to prevent PPH and due to its relative low cost, ease of administration and storage at room temperature, it may be of particular use in developing countries. It is administered rectally in a dose of 800mcg as a single dose. It can also be used for induction of labour.

Chapter 4

Monitoring the mother

Dermot Nicolson, Rachel Collis

'Safe anaesthesia does not require a mass of complex equipment; the greatest degree of safety for the available resources will be achieved by a careful, conscientious anaesthetist who balances risk, benefit and cost in the context in which he or she works.'

(Runciman 1993)

> **Key points**
> - Monitoring aims to improve patient safety
> - The most important monitor is the trained anaesthetist or anaesthetic practitioner
> - Knowledge of the benefits and limitations of each monitor is important
> - Fetal monitoring is an important part of intrapartum care.

4.1 Basic principles

Monitoring consists of continuous clinical observation and electronic surveillance of the patient, so that any deviation from normal can be detected early, corrected appropriately, and harm to the patient prevented. Monitoring will not prevent all adverse events, but should reduce their incidence by giving early warning. The World Federation of Societies of Anaesthesiology adopted standards (International Task Force on Anaesthesia Safety 1993) on the safe practice of anaesthesia. Many countries have developed their own standards for monitoring that are suitable for the level of resources available to them. All published guidelines state that the most important monitor of all is the trained anaesthetist continuously observing the patient. The source of most critical incidents during anaesthesia have been identified as hypoxic gas mixtures, gas flows, breathing systems, tracheal tubes, the airway, and ventilation. The International Standards for Safe Practice of Anaesthesia recommended that an oxygen supply failure alarm, an oxygen analyser, pulse oximeter, capnograph, and electrocardiograph be used for all anaesthetics. Some of these monitors may not be affordable in many countries. Therefore, the priority sequence for monitor acquisition in areas with limited resources should be a stethoscope, sphygmomanometer (blood pressure cuff and pressure gauge), oxygen analyser if nitrous oxide is used, pulse oximeter, capnograph and ventilator alarms. An ECG, a defibrillator, a spirometer, and a thermometer should also be available.

Basic Principles of Monitoring

- The most important monitor is the trained anaesthetist
- Best method of monitoring should be determined by good preoperative assessment of the patient
- Equipment should be checked prior to anaesthesia
- Appropriate alarm limits should be set prior to anaesthesia
- Monitoring must be started before induction and continued into the recovery period
- The concentration of oxygen in the inspired gas should be verified, at least at the start of each anaesthetic session
- Patient oxygenation should be monitored clinically by visual observation and the use of a pulse oximeter is highly recommended
- Adequate airway and ventilation should be continuously monitored by observation and auscultation whenever practicable
- A capnograph is highly recommended for confirmation of the correct placement of the tracheal tube and the adequacy of ventilation
- A disconnection alarm should be used whenever mechanical ventilation is employed
- The circulation should be monitored continuously by palpation of the pulse, auscultation of the heart and augmented with a pulse oximeter, if possible
- Blood pressure should be measured at least every 5 minutes.
- Continuous monitoring of heart rate by electrocardiograph is highly recommended
- A written record of the details provided by monitoring devices and clinical observation should be kept
- The same standards of monitoring apply when regional/local anaesthesia and sedation are used
- Fetal monitoring is an important part of intra-partum care.

4.2 Monitoring the mother

4.2.1 The anaesthetist as monitor

An anaesthetic practitioner must be present throughout anaesthesia using clinical skills and monitors to care for the patient continuously. During anaesthesia, the patient's physiological state and depth of anaesthesia (general anaesthesia) need continual assessment.

4.2.1.1 Cardiovascular system

The cardiovascular system provides oxygenated blood to the tissues. A good cardiac output is likely to be present if there is a strong regular pulse, normal skin colour, warm fingers and a urine output of >0.5 ml/kg/hr. A capillary refill time of <2 seconds also suggests normal cardiac output and good tissue perfusion. Palpation of the pulse gives information on the heart rate and rhythm. When the pulse is weak and thready, it indicates a low blood pressure.

4.2.1.2 Respiratory system

Adequate ventilation and oxygenation must be monitored continuously. Observation of the patient's colour, movement of the chest and breathing system reservoir bag are essential. Tissue oxygenation should be monitored by visual examination with adequate illumination and exposure of the patient should be ensured. Cyanosis is an important sign but can be difficult to detect until hypoxaemia is severe. It is best looked for in the mucous membranes and the colour of the blood in the surgical field. If cyanosis is detected, the cause or fault needs to be recognised and corrected immediately. When the anaesthetized patient is breathing spontaneously, signs of airway obstruction include tracheal tug, paradoxical chest movement and failure of the reservoir bag to move. Bilateral equal chest movement and auscultation of the chest confirms the position of the tracheal tube.

4.2.1.3 Consciousness

Awareness is a complication of general anaesthesia. Signs of light anaesthesia are those of sympathetic activity: sweating, tachycardia, hypertension, pallor, and pupil dilatation.

4.2.2 Stethoscope

The stethoscope is simple, cheap and can be used to monitor both the respiratory and circulatory systems. It gives information on heart rate, heart sounds and presence of murmurs. Chest auscultation gives information on lung air entry and added sounds. It is useful to aid in the diagnosis of oesophageal or endo-bronchial intubation.

4.2.3 Blood pressure monitoring

Blood pressure (BP) should be measured every 5 minutes or more frequently if clinically indicated. Methods for BP measurement include palpatory, auscultatory, oscillometric, and direct invasive BP monitoring.

4.2.3.1 *Palpatory method*

This method involves inflating a BP cuff (sphygmomanometer) on the upper arm and palpating the radial pulse at the same time. The cuff is inflated until the pulse disappears and then slowly deflated. The pressure at which the radial pulse returns is the systolic BP.

4.2.3.2 *Auscultatory method*

This method involves inflating a cuff on the upper arm to a pressure above systolic pressure and listening over the brachial artery in the ante-cubital fossa as the cuff is slowly deflated. The five Korotkoff sounds are heard on deflation:

Phase I – The first appearance of tapping sounds
Phase II – A blowing or swishing sound
Phase III – The return of sharp tapping sounds (softer than phase I)
Phase IV – A softer blowing sound that disappears
Phase V – The point when all sounds disappear

Phase I represents systolic BP and Phase IV or V can be used to identify diastolic BP. **During pregnancy it is recommended that Phase V be used to identify diastolic BP.**

4.2.3.3 *Oscillometric method*

This is an automated method of BP measurement. The anaesthetist sets how often the BP is measured (usually every 3–5 minutes) and the cuff automatically inflates and deflates. As it deflates, pressure oscillations in the cuff are sensed by a pressure transducer and stored electronically. Systolic and diastolic pressures are estimated when the amplitude of oscillations rapidly increase and decrease respectively. A mean blood pressure reading is also given, which occurs when the oscillation amplitude is greatest.

4.2.4 **Electrocardiogram**

The electrocardiogram (ECG) is a continuous recording of the electrical activity of the heart, which is measured at the skin surface with three electrodes. The ECG provides information on the heart rate, the presence of arrhythmias, conduction defects and any degree of cardiac ischaemia. Electrical cardiac activity can still occur in the absence of a cardiac output, for example severe hypovolaemia or cardiac tamponade, which limits its use as a monitor.

4.2.5 **Pulse oximeter**

The pulse oximeter is considered to be one of greatest advances in patient monitoring. It measures and gives a continuous reading of haemoglobin oxygen saturation, and is therefore a cyanosis monitor. The pulse oximeter allows the detection of unsuspected arterial hypoxaemia when clinical assessment reveals no abnormality, allowing treatment before damage to the patient occurs. The probe is

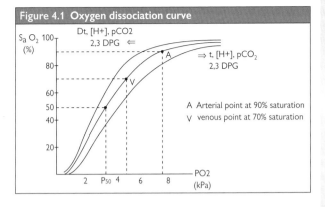

Figure 4.1 Oxygen dissociation curve

$S_a O_2$ 100 (%)

Dt, [H+], pCO2
2,3 DPG ⇐

⇒ t, [H+], pCO_2
2,3 DPG

A Arterial point at 90% saturation
V venous point at 70% saturation

PO_2 (kPa)

usually placed on the patients' finger and works by measuring changes in light absorption. It is a powerful monitoring tool in theatre, recovery, intensive care and for transferring critically ill patients.

Although the pulse oximeter is invaluable, it does have some limitations. A fall in oxygen saturation occurs after a decrease in arterial oxygen tension. However, due to the shape of the oxyhaemoglobin dissociation curve, there must be a large fall in oxygen tension to produce a measurable fall in oxygen saturation, especially between 90 and 100% O_2 saturation. Saturations <95% are abnormal (Figure 4.1).

The pulse oximeter may give inaccurate results from movement artefact, low peripheral perfusion, electrical interference, coloured nail polish and it is not accurate when saturations fall below 50%. The presence of carboxyhaemoglobin in the blood will give a falsely high result and methaemoglobin will result in a falsely low result. If methylene blue is injected IV, it will result in a low reading for a few minutes.

4.2.6 **Capnography**

A capnograph gives a continuous and pictorial display of CO_2 concentration. It gives a breath-by-breath measurement of end-tidal CO_2, which is closely related to the arterial partial pressure of CO_2 (Figure 4.2). The capnograph gives early warning of many life-threatening situations making it an extremely useful monitor during general anaesthesia. The absence of a trace could indicate oesophageal intubation, disconnection of the breathing system, tracheal tube displacement or circulatory arrest. A low or falling end-tidal CO_2 trace could indicate hyperventilation, pulmonary embolus (thrombus or gas) or decreased cardiac output. A high reading or rising end-tidal CO_2 could indicate inadequate ventilation, re-breathing of CO_2 if the baseline does not return to zero, or malignant hyperthermia. A slow upstroke and rising plateaux indicate airway obstruction e.g. asthma, COPD or bronchospasm (Figure 4.3).

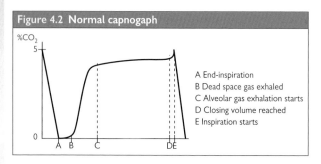

Figure 4.2 Normal capnogaph

%CO$_2$

A End-inspiration
B Dead space gas exhaled
C Alveolar gas exhalation starts
D Closing volume reached
E Inspiration starts

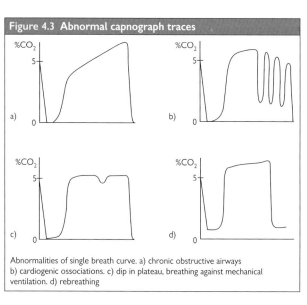

Figure 4.3 Abnormal capnograph traces

%CO$_2$

a)

%CO$_2$

b)

%CO$_2$

c)

%CO$_2$

d)

Abnormalities of single breath curve. a) chronic obstructive airways
b) cardiogenic ossociations. c) dip in plateau, breathing against mechanical
ventilation. d) rebreathing

4.2.7 Ventilator alarms

Ventilator alarms should be used during positive pressure ventilation
to guard against patient disconnections, gas leaks, obstruction, or
ventilation malfunction. Capnographs, pressure sensors, and volume
monitors can all be used as disconnection monitors.

4.2.7.1 Pressure monitoring

A pressure monitor has a sensor placed in the inspiratory limb of the
ventilator system, from where the peak inspiratory pressure is measured. A decrease or increase in pressure activates the alarm. Causes

of a low pressure include disconnection, a gas leak or inadequate fresh gas flow. An increase in pressure could be due to obstruction in the ventilator tubing or in the patient's airway.

4.2.7.2 *Volume monitoring*

These take the form of respirometers or flow sensors, and they are usually placed in the expiratory limb of the breathing circuit. They measure tidal volume and/or minute ventilation.

4.2.8 **Documentation**

Good documentation helps to improve patient care and an accurate anaesthetic record must always be kept. It should include the preoperative assessment, description of the anaesthetic technique, intraoperative vital signs obtained from clinical examination and monitors, and postoperative instructions. Vital signs should be recorded at 5 minute intervals as trends will then become evident and any adverse trends may be corrected before any harm comes to the patient.

Chapter 5

Basic principles of obstetric anaesthesia

Dermot Nicolson, Rachel Collis

Key points

- A pregnant woman is at increased risk of regurgitation and aspiration, especially if general anaesthesia is performed
- Antacids must be administered to high risk women in labour and prior to emergency or elective caesarean section (CS)
- Pregnant women should never lie completely supine
- Aorto-caval compression can be minimized by placing the mother in 15° left lateral tilt during CS
- The choice of anaesthetic technique is dependent on the urgency of delivery, maternal well-being and the mother's wishes.

5.1 Antacid prophylaxis

Regurgitation and inhalation of gastric contents during general anaesthesia can result in pneumonitis, with considerable risk of maternal morbidity or death. Pregnant women are at particular risk of aspiration because of reduced effectiveness of the lower oesophageal sphincter, increased intragastric pressure caused by the large uterus and delayed gastric emptying if opiates are used during labour. The increased risk of aspiration starts from 16–18 weeks gestation and continues into the first week postpartum. The risk of aspiration is reduced by: avoidance of general anaesthesia (GA) and increased use of regional anaesthesia, decreasing the volume of stomach contents and increasing gastric pH, and prevention of regurgitation if GA is used.

5.1.1 Reduction of gastric volume

During labour, solid food should be limited, and all women for elective caesarean section must be starved for 6 hours prior to surgery.

The prokinetic drug, metoclopramide, increases gastric emptying and can be administered IV to reduce gastric volume prior to emergency and elective CS. It is particularly important prior to a general anaesthetic being performed.

5.1.2 Reduction of gastric pH

Gastric pH can be reduced with antacids (e.g. sodium citrate) H_2 receptor antagonists (e.g. ranitidine) and proton pump inhibitors (e.g. omeprazole). There is limited evidence to support the routine use of acid prophylaxis during normal labour. However, mothers at high risk of surgical intervention may benefit from oral administration of regular H_2 receptor antagonists, which are relatively inexpensive and safe.

Guidelines for pharmacological aspiration prevention

Normal low risk labour
- No prophylaxis

High risk labour
- Ranitidine 150mg PO 6 hourly

Elective caesarean section
- Ranitidine 150mg PO the night before surgery
- Ranitidine 150mg PO the morning of surgery
- +/− Metoclopramide 10mg IV/PO immediately pre surgery

Emergency caesarean section
- Ranitidine 50mg IV, +/− metoclopramide 10mg IV
- 30 ml Sodium citrate 0.3M PO immediately prior to GA

5.1.3 Prevention of regurgitation

A rapid sequence induction of anaesthesia, with the application of cricoid pressure during induction of GA, will prevent the passive regurgitation of stomach contents until the airway is secured with a cuffed tracheal tube.

5.2 Managing aorto-caval compression

Pregnant women should never lie completely supine, as the gravid uterus will cause compression of the inferior vena cava, leading to a decrease in cardiac output, followed by profound hypotension, and compression of the abdominal aorta, leading to reduced placental perfusion and fetal compromise. Aorto-caval compression can be minimized by altering the maternal position, therefore releasing the pressure placed on the vena cava and aorta by the gravid uterus (Fig 5.1).

5.2.1 **Full lateral position**

This is the most effective position for relieving aorto-caval compression but is not practical when performing a CS. Following regional anaesthesia, the woman should be placed in the full lateral position if hypotension occurs, until the blood pressure returns to normal.

5.2.2 **15° left lateral tilt**

A 15° left lateral tilt is the commonest position for operative procedures when the mother is on a moveable operating table. This position only partially removes aorto-caval compression; however, it is a compromise as CS is still possible.

5.2.3 **Wedge**

The uterus is displaced by placing a wedge (a pillow or rolled up blanket can be used) under the mother's right hip. This is useful if the mother is lying on a surface, which cannot tilt, such as a delivery bed.

5.2.4 **Manual uterine displacement**

The uterus is manually displaced to the left by an assistant. This is effective but is usually only a temporary measure.

5.3 **Anaesthetic techniques**

When deciding on an anaesthetic technique, consideration should be given to the indication for CS, the urgency of the surgery, the health of the mother and fetus, and the mothers' wishes.

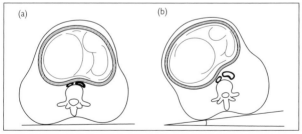

Figure 5.1 Aorto-caval compression. (a) In the supine position, blood flow through the vena cava and aorta is significantly reduced, causing maternal and fetal compromise. The efficacy of left lateral displacement was demonstrated in 1972. The full left or right lateral position completely relieves aorto-caval compression. (b) Elevating the mother's hip 10–15cm completely relieves aorto-caval compression in 58% of term parturients.

5.3.1 **Regional anaesthesia**

5.3.1.1 Spinal anaesthesia

Spinal anaesthesia is appropriate for most elective and urgent CS in mothers without an epidural in-situ. The advantages of spinal anaesthesia are its simplicity of insertion, rapid onset of action and dense neural blockade. Immediate bonding between mother and newborn is another advantage.

5.3.1.2 Epidural anaesthesia

An epidural sited for labour analgesia can be topped-up if an urgent CS is required. Incremental LA doses via the epidural catheter may be titrated to achieve the desired level of sensory block and will usually result in less hypotension compared to a spinal anaesthestic. However, the speed of onset of sensory block is slower, which is a disadvantage when delivery is very urgent, and the density and quality of sensory block may be less than a spinal anaesthetic.

5.3.1.3 Combined spinal epidural (CSE)

A CSE offers the rapid onset and dense sensory block of a spinal anaesthetic, combined with the versatility of an epidural catheter which can be topped-up to prolong anaesthesia as required. The epidural component may also be used for postoperative analgesia.

Absolute contraindications to regional anaesthesia
• Maternal refusal
• Localized infection at the insertion site or generalized sepsis
• Full patient anticoagulation or coagulation abnormalities
• True allergy to local anaesthetic—very rare.

5.3.2 **General anaesthesia (GA)**

GA is indicated if immediate delivery is necessary. It has the advantage of the shortest onset of anaesthesia to delivery time. There are few absolute contraindications to GA, but it should be avoided in patients with a known or predicted difficult airway, a history of malignant hyperthermia and in patients with severe respiratory disease. The disadvantages of GA are an increased risk of maternal aspiration and the potential increased risk of difficult intubation in pregnant women. The anaesthetist and surgeon must always weigh up the severity of fetal distress against the maternal risk of GA.

Chapter 6

Pain relief in labour

Eleanor Lewis, Sarah Harries

Key points

- The pain of labour is severe
- Effective pain relief in labour is not only humane, but has immense psychological and physical benefits for both mother and baby
- Fear and isolation can increase a woman's perception of pain during labour and can adversely affect outcome
- A wide variety of psychological and pharmacological methods of analgesia can be offered to reduce pain
- All opiates cross the placenta and may precipitate neonatal respiratory depression at birth
- Epidural analgesia is the most effective form of labour analgaesia in reducing maternal pain, cardiovascular work, and anxiety.

6.1 Pain pathways

During the first stage of labour, pain is caused by uterine contractions and progressive dilatation of the cervix. It is transmitted from the uterus and cervix via afferent nerve fibres to enter the spinal cord via T10, T11, T12 and L1 spinal nerves (see Figure 6.1). During the second stage of labour, pain is caused by uterine contractions and in addition, stretching of the birth canal and perineum. The latter additional pain impulses are conveyed via S2 to S4 spinal nerves.

6.2 Effects of pain on maternal physiology

Labour pain causes profound effects on maternal cardio-respiratory physiology, as well as maternal distress and intense fatigue. During labour, maternal catecholamine levels e.g. adrenaline, are increased, leading to a 25–50% rise in the cardiac output (CO). In addition, 300–500 ml of blood is displaced from the uterus into the central

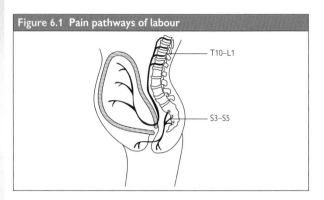

Figure 6.1 Pain pathways of labour

T10–L1

S3–S5

circulation with each contraction, which further increases the CO. This is of particular importance to the parturient with significant cardiac disease. Increased catecholamines also cause maternal hyperglycemia and lipolysis which can contribute to fetal acidosis, and they also have a tocolytic effect on the uterus, thereby contributing to dysfunctional labour. It may also harm the fetus because intense painful contractions cause an increase in maternal minute ventilation of up to 3 times, leading to a decrease in $PaCO_2$ to < 3 kPa, which shifts the maternal oxyhaemoglobin dissociation curve to the left causing less oxygen to be released to the fetus. The fetus is at risk of hypoxia and hypercapnia. On the other hand, maternal hypocapnia causes vasoconstriction and reduced uterine blood flow which can lead to fetal acidosis and distress. The effect of pain on other systems are summarised in Table 6.1. Therefore, providing effective analgesia in labour reduces these undesired effects of pain on both mother and baby.

6.3 **Non-pharmacological analgesia**

There is a wide spectrum of options available for pain relief in labour. In rural areas, deliveries may be supervised by traditional birth attendants who may practice labour analgesia in a non-standardized fashion. However, despite effective options being made available, many women prefer to avoid pharmacological or invasive methods of pain relief. Non pharmacological options can be grouped into psychological, physical and others:

6.3.1 **Psychological therapies**

Wide variations in mother: birthing attendant ratios exist; however, a 1:1 ratio is considered ideal. Unfortunately, this ratio is difficult to

Table 6.1 Physiological response to labour pain	
System	**Response to pain**
CVS	Pain increases catecholamines levels leading to tachycardia, increase contractility and increase systemic vascular resistance. All increase myocardial oxygen demand.
Placenta	Pain increases catecholamines levels leading to vasoconstriction of umbilical vessels and consequently reducing placental blood flow.
Respiratory	Pain increase minute ventilation resulting in maternal hypocapnoea. The consequent respiratory alkalosis shifts the haemoglobin-oxygen dissociation curve to the left thereby reducing oxygen off-loading to the fetus.
GIT	Pain reduces gastric emptying, therefore increasing the risk of aspiration.

attain in many circumstances, leading to parturients labouring unattended for long lengths of time. It is well recognized that isolation adversely affects a mother's experience of labour.

6.3.1.1 Emotional support

Emotional support is essential to a satisfying childbirth experience.

A Cochrane review involving 13,000 women from 11 different countries showed that women who had the continuous presence of a supportive companion, e.g. husband, relative or friend during labour, had slightly shorter labours, reduced requirement for analgesia and were more likely to have spontaneous vaginal deliveries. These women reported greater satisfaction with the entire childbirth experience. This feeling was true despite large cultural differences, obstetric practices and environmental conditions.

Continuous support was associated with the greatest benefits when the provider was not a member of the hospital staff, when it began early in labour and in settings in which epidural analgesia was not routinely available. This resource is widely available, especially in communities where extended families are common. It does not increase costs and is useful at any stage of labour. Unfortunately, the presence of husbands or relatives in the delivery room is actively discouraged in many public hospitals. A keen commitment to changing this practice will overcome many of the existing obstacles.

6.3.1.2 Mind-body interventions

The Lamaze technique is one of the commonly encountered methods. The woman is educated prior to labour on the use of breathing, relaxation, meditation and visualization techniques to decrease pain perception. Hypnosis may have a calming effect during labour; however, only ~20–25% of labouring women are susceptible.

6.3.1.3 Physical therapies

Massage

The use of massage to soothe the individual and release tension is an old practice. Based on the 'gate control' theory of pain, massage may reduce pain transmission, thereby helping to relieve labour pain. Massage may also relieve pain by improving blood flow and oxygenation of tissues.

Transcutaneous electrical nerve stimulation (TENS)

A low voltage electrical impulse is delivered to the skin via four pads which are placed over the lower back with a 'boost' during uterine contractions. Its mechanism of action is also based on the 'gate control' theory of pain. There is no strong evidence to support the efficacy of TENS analgesia; however, it is simple to use and has no adverse effects on the mother or fetus and allows the mother to mobilize freely. Its efficacy is probably greatest when used in the latent or early phase of labour.

Hydrotherapy

Immersion in warm water during labour has been shown to reduce other analgesia requirements and operative delivery rates. The popularity of birthing pools is increasing in some countries, e.g. the United Kingdom.

Acupuncture

Fine needles are inserted into specific body points to relieve pain. Acupuncture has been shown to relieve labour pain in some studies but more evidence is required to advocate its use.

6.3.1.4 Others

Herbal extracts

For many women, the herbal practitioner is readily available and more importantly is often more affordable. Parturients may have taken a variety of herbal mixtures prescribed in a non-standardized fashion. This is more common when there is a preceding history of infertility or a history of obstetric difficulty. Women may be reluctant to admit what herbs have been prescribed, which is a problem as they may precipitate unexplained or unexpected reactions to conventional drugs or therapies. It is largely accepted that that the herbalist is an inescapable reality of health practice in the developing world.

Aromatherapy

Essential plant oils can be massaged into the skin, or inhaled using a steam infusion or burner. The mechanism of action is unclear. Studies have demonstrated psychological improvement in mood and anxiety levels.

6.4 **Pharmacological analgesia for labour**

Intravenous, intramuscular and inhalation analgesia can provide useful pain relief to mothers where regional analgesia is either contra-indicated or not available. Systemic opiates are the most widely used drugs for labour analgesia. Ketamine may also have a useful function. Inhalation agents include 50:50 oxygen/nitrous oxide mix (Entonox®) and low dose inhalation anaesthetics.

6.4.1 **Opiate analgesia**

Pethidine—is widely used in the UK as a first line drug for labour analgesia. It is usually administered intramuscularly in two divided doses of 75mg every 4 hours. Its onset time is within 10 minutes when given IM, and lasts for 2–3 hours. It readily crosses the placenta and ionizes in the relative acidic fetal circulation, leading to accumulation. Peak fetal concentrations occur 2–3 hours after maternal administration.

The effects include analgesia, amnesia, dysphoria, and sedation. Side effects include maternal and neonatal respiratory depression, nausea, sedation and hallucinations. It is metabolized to norpethidine which has pro-convulsant properties, therefore it should be used with caution in patients with PET, renal failure or uncontrolled epilepsy.

Morphine—Morphine 5–10mg may be administered IM or IV as an incremental bolus dose or via a patient controlled analgesia pump. It is effective in providing analgesia, amnesia and euphoria. Its peak analgesic effect is 30–60 minutes after IM administration and lasts for 3–4 hours. It rapidly crosses the placenta but diffuses back into the maternal circulation. Side effects include nausea and respiratory depression, which limit its use.

Fentanyl —This is a highly potent synthetic opiate, which acts within 2–5 minutes after IV administration of doses 25–100mcg which can be effective for up to 30–60 minutes. It is highly lipid soluble and readily crosses the placenta. It is a potent respiratory depressant, so both the mother and baby need to be monitored closely in the intra-partum and post-natal period

6.4.2 **Non opiate analgesics**

Ketamine—Ketamine is not used in the developed world for labour analgesia; however, it can be a useful, short acting analgesic in settings where it is available. Following an IV bolus dose of 0.1mg/kg ketamine, an IV infusion of 0.2mg/kg/hr may be continued, titrated to effect. Ketamine does not cause maternal respiratory depression; however, nausea, dizziness and hallucinations are common side effects. It should be used with caution in mothers with pregnancy-induced hypertension or PET. Neonatal depression occurs at IV doses of >2mg/kg.

6.4.3 Inhalational analgaesia

50:50 mix of oxygen/nitrous oxide (Entonox®) is used by >90% of labouring mothers in the UK. It has limited analgesic effects, but its dissociation and relaxation properties improve the mothers' perception of labour pain. It is available in cylinders, which are blue with white shoulders and can be administered by either a mouth piece incorporating a one way valve, or a face mask. Entonox diffuses freely across alveolar membranes to provide rapid effects with minimal accumulation but 15% of mothers will experience nausea. It may be teratogenic in early pregnancy and there is a theoretical risk of bone marrow suppression with prolonged use.

Volatile agents—low inspired concentrations of isoflurane (0.75%) or sevoflurane (0.8%) may be used in oxygen: air or Entonox® mixtures to provide analgesia. Their use is limited by maternal sedation and loss of airway reflexes. At low concentrations, Apgar scores are unaffected.

6.5 Regional analgesia for labour

Regional analgesia is the most effective form of labour analgesia. It reduces maternal pain, cardiovascular work and anxiety, with minimal effects on the fetus. In addition, a 'working' epidural for labour can reduce the need for general anaesthesia if operative delivery or post-delivery surgery is required. Regional analgesia can be achieved with either an epidural, single-shot spinal or a combined spinal-epidural technique.

For details of these techniques, refer to Chapters 7 and 8.

6.5.1 Indications for regional analgesia for labour

Regional analgesia is widely available in the developed world and has changed the labour experience for many women, making it much more pleasurable and satisfying. Increasing maternal education in the developing world is creating a greater awareness of choice for labour analgesia in these settings, therefore requests for these options will continue to increase in the future. See Table 6.2.

Contraindications to regional techniques are detailed in Chapter 7.

6.5.2 Pre-requisites to establishing a regional technique

Before any regional technique is established, there must be appropriately trained staff and equipment to perform the procedure, and subsequently monitor the patients' vital signs and fetal heart rate (CTG) for the duration of epidural analgesia or spinal block.

Table 6.2 Indications for regional analgesia in labour

Maternal request	Adequate analgesia in labour is not only humane but has immense psychological and physical benefits for both mother and baby. Regional techniques have been shown to provide the most effective pain relief in labour.
Pre-eclampsia	To optimize BP control
Augmentation or Induction of Labour	Augmenting labour with a oxytocin infusion increases the frequency and intensity of contractions, and the incidence of operative delivery
Maternal cardiac or respiratory disease	To minimize the effects of circulating catecholamines on cardiac work and aid haemodynamic stability To reduce the increase in minute ventilation associated with labour and delivery
Predicted difficult airway or general anaesthesia	An effective epidural established in early labour may reduce the risks associated with GA—difficult ventilation/intubation in morbid obesity or PET Anaesthetic reactions in MH-susceptible patients or suxamethonium apnoea
Occipito-posterior presentation	Often associated with increased pain during labour and greater incidence of operative delivery

Wide bore IV access must be established before the regional technique, to enable prompt administration of drugs in the event of maternal hypotension or collapse. Full resuscitation facilities must be checked and immediately available, with a means of administering oxygen.

6.5.3 **Information and consent**

Any explanation regarding the planned procedure should be tailored to the individual patient, without compromising the basic principles of consent. The aim is to inform without inducing unnecessary fear.

Essential information should include: basic description of the procedure, the correct position and the need to keep as still as possible, risk of failure or ineffective block, nausea and vomiting, need for blood pressure monitoring, tenderness or bruising at the insertion site and the risk of severe headache following accidental dural puncture i.e. ~1% for an experienced operator.

The patient may request further information about the rare but severe consequences of epidural and spinal placement. The risk of infection, e.g. epidural abscess requiring surgery, meningitis or the risk of neurological complications, e.g. paralysis, nerve damage, have an incidence of ~ 1:10,000 when practiced under strict aseptic conditions.

Following the procedure, document your technique and any complications accurately on the anaesthetic chart.

6.5.4 **Insertion technique**

The ideal inter-vertebral spaces for epidural catheter insertion for labour analgesia are between T12 and L5. For details of the equipment required, patient positioning and the technique of insertion, see Chapter 8.

6.5.5 **Drugs that can be used in the epidural space**

The most common group of drugs that are used for epidural analgesia are local anaesthetics and opiates.

6.5.5.1 *Local anaesthetics (LA)*

LA causes reversible blockade of action potential transmission in nerve fibres, preferentially blocking small C and Aδ fibres, followed by larger Aα and B fibres. LA in the epidural space principally acts by diffusing across the dura into the CSF, and thus into nerve roots and the spinal cord. LA toxicity leads to serious central nervous system effects followed by cardiovascular collapse and death. Signs of serious toxicity progressively include; extensive numbness and loss of motor power, tingling around the mouth, slurred speech, tinnitus, agitation, convulsions, loss of consciousness, cardiovascular collapse, respiratory depression, death.

6.5.5.2 *Opiates*

Opiates bind to μ receptors in the substantia gelatinosa of the spinal cord, blocking pain transmission. Epidural opiates diffuse across the dura into the substantia gelationosa. In addition, opiates are absorbed into the epidural veins and are absorbed systemically. Common side effects include nausea, pruritis, urinary retention and respiratory depression. Delayed respiratory depression can occur up to 6–8 hours after spinal fentanyl and up to 24 hours after morphine. The main benefits of epidural opiates are that they improve the quality of the sensory block, therefore reducing the need for larger doses of local anaesthetics.

6.5.6 **Pudendal nerve block**

It is possible for a pudendal nerve block to be sited on each side of the birth canal to provide analgesia for the second stage of labour or a straightforward instrumental delivery. The pudendal nerve arises from the sacral plexus (S2–S4) and supplies the perineum, vulva and vagina. This technique is usually performed by the obstetrician via a transvaginal approach. With the patient in lithotomy position, the ischial spine is palpated from within the vagina. A long guarded needle is inserted ~1.5cm beyond the ischial spine and the sacrospinal ligament. After negative aspiration of blood, 10 ml of 0.25% or 0.5% bupivacaine is infiltrated bilaterally. Unfortunately, the success rate of achieving effective analgesia is low, as too often there is limited time to allow the local anaesthetic solution to be effective due to the urgency of the situation.

Table 6.3 Suggested dosing regimes

Technique	Drugs and their doses
Epidural	10 ml 0.1% bupivacaine + 2mcg/ml fentanyl (test dose)
	Followed by further 10–20 ml of same mixture to establish sensory block from T8–S5
	Maintenance options:
	10 ml 0.1% bupivacaine + 2mcg/ml fentanyl every hour by bolus dose or via infusion device
	PCEA regime – 0.1% bupivacaine + 2mcg/ml fentanyl background infusion 0–6 ml/hour, 5 ml bolus dose every 10–20 minutes
Spinal	3–5 ml 0.1% bupivacaine +/– 2mcg/ml fentanyl
	1ml 0.5% heavy bupivacaine +/– 5–10mcg fentanyl
	A low dose, single-shot, spinal technique provides almost immediate labour analgesia for ~60 minutes. This may be sufficient time for a multiparous woman to deliver or time for an epidural to be sited if labour is prolonged.
Combined spinal & epidural technique (CSE)	CSE dosing as for isolated spinal and epidural techniques, see above.
	As a combined technique, it offers the advantages of immediate analgesia from the spinal component and maintenance epidural analgesia. No drugs should be administered via the epidural catheter until the spinal sensory block has started to recede and the first dose should be the suggested test dose as above.

If suturing of the perineum is required after a pudendal nerve block and a successful instrumental delivery, local infiltration of the labia with local anaesthetic is still required.

Chapter 7

Spinal anaesthesia

Paul Clyburn

Key points

- Where spinal anaesthesia can be safely performed, it is the method of choice for caesarean section in most situations
- It should not be used when there is haemodynamic instability such as hypovolaemia from haemorrhage (obvious or concealed), or significant stenotic heart valve lesions
- It should not be used in patients with bleeding disorders, including those on effective anticoagulant therapy
- Strict asepsis should be used when performing spinal anaesthesia
- Position the patient carefully (with good back flexion and avoid twisting of the spine) BEFORE scrubbing up to perform the block
- Full equipment to undertake general anaesthesia should be available together with monitoring of pulse and blood pressure, resuscitation drugs and vasoconstrictor drugs to treat the hypotension that frequently occurs
- Following spinal anaesthesia, the mother should be placed in a left tilted or pelvis wedged position to reduce the effects of aorto caval compression
- Following surgery, the mother should be monitored in the same way as following a general anaesthetic.

Spinal anaesthesia is a safe and popular technique for caesarean section. It can also be used for other obstetric procedures such as: perineal suturing and repairs, evacuation of a retained placenta and forceps delivery. It avoids complications associated with general anaesthesia in pregnancy such as acid aspiration syndrome and failed intubation. It allows the mother to be awake, see and care for her newborn baby and gives good pain relief to the mother in the first few hours after the operation. Unlike a general anaesthetic, the baby is not sedated by the drugs administered to the mother. Finally, it is cheap, easy to perform and suitable for most patients.

You should not give spinal anaesthesia to, or at least exercise caution in:

- A mother who refuses the technique
- A mother who is shocked from blood or fluid loss
- A mother with major heart valve problems, especially those with stenotic valves
- Patients with bleeding disorders (patients with hypertensive disease of pregnancy should have their platelet and clotting function checked)
- A patient with localized sepsis at the intended injection site or major systemic infection.
- Patients suspected of having raised intracranial pressure.

7.1 **Anatomy and mechanism of action**

The spinal cord is the main nerve pathway from the brain to the rest of the body and is contained within the vertebral canal, made up of 24 vertebrae, which make up the backbone. The spinal cord is surrounded by the dural membrane forming a sac, which contains cerebrospinal fluid (CSF). The spinal cord gives off pairs of segmental nerves, which leave the spinal canal between each adjacent vertebra to supply much of the body. The spinal cord ends in adults at around the 1st and 2nd lumbar vertebra but the dural sac extends lower to the sacrum, so that a needle inserted into the sac below the 2nd lumbar vertebra should not damage the spinal cord.

Local anaesthetic agents injected into the spinal sac below the 2nd lumbar vertebra will spread in the CSF and block nerve transmission along the spinal nerves. The number of spinal nerves blocked above the place of insertion will depend upon the extent of spread of local anaesthetic in the spinal sac. This spread is determined by: the amount of drug administered, whether the drug solution is more or less dense than CSF and the position of the patient following insertion i.e. denser solutions being heavier will tend to go to the more dependant parts of the spinal sac, whilst with less dense 'light' solutions, the converse occurs. Barbotage, a process where the local anaesthetic is part injected and then CSF drawn back into the syringe mixing it with the drug remaining in the syringe and then reinjected, also increases the spread of local anaesthetic.

Spinal nerves are mixed nerves and contain both sensory and motor nerve fibres. In the thoracic region, they also contain the sympathetic nerves supplying much of the body. When sympathetic nerves are blocked by local anaesthetics, there is a relaxation of vascular smooth muscle which normally requires sympathetic nerves to maintain their tone. This relaxation produces vasodilatation and a tendency to hypotension. This effect is greater in the supine pregnant patient as vasoconstriction is important to overcome compression of the vena cava (and aorta) by the pregnant uterus, which reduces flow back to the heart and leads to a reduction in cardiac output. This is known as aorto-caval compression. To counteract this effect, it is important that **following spinal anaesthesia, the mother is never placed flat on her back but is tilted to the left (ideally 15°) to minimize compression of the aorta and vena cava by the gravid uterus.**

7.2 **Preparation**

The mother should be given a full explanation about the benefits of spinal anaesthesia, as well as how it will be carried out and what she should expect during the operation. She should be told that very quickly she will experience warmth and 'pins and needles' over her lower body, find her legs become heavy and that she may not be able to move them, that she may feel light headed and occasionally develop nausea and may vomit.

Although spinal anaesthesia avoids general anaesthesia, all equipment to give a general anaesthetic should be available. If the spinal anaesthetic doesn't work or if there are difficulties with the block or surgery, a general anaesthetic may have to be given quickly and everything should be ready for such a possibility. For the same reason, the patient should have identical pre-operative preparation as regards antacid prophylaxis as for a general anaesthetic (see Chapter 12).

7.2.1 **Equipment**

You will need the following:

- Suitable clean work surface
- Sterile dressing pack with swabs and forceps (for cleaning)
- Range of suitable sized syringes and needles for local anaesthetic infiltration
- Sterile drapes able to surround the area of insertion
- Sterile spinal needle—ideally 24–27 gauge pencil point
- Spinal drugs
- 1% plain lidocaine for skin infiltration
- Vasopressor—see below
- Ideally a particle filter needle for drawing up intrathecal drugs

Because of the tendency for hypotension, it is essential that a large bore (at least 16 gauge) intravenous cannula is inserted into a good vein and attached to a fluid infusion so that fluids and drugs can be administered quickly to treat any hypotension. A vasoconstrictor drug should be prepared ready to administer and treat maternal hypotension and bradycardia. Suggested vasopressor drugs include:

- Ephedrine diluted in saline to give 3–5mg/ml
- Methoxamine diluted to 2mg/ml
- Phenylephrine diluted to 25–50mcg/ml
- Metaraminol diluted 1mg/ml
- Adrenaline diluted to 25–50mcg/ml or noradrenaline diluted to 20mcg/ml

All the above dilutions should be given 1 ml at a time and titrated to effect. Ephedrine is most commonly used but there is increasing evidence that phenylephrine is a better drug to use if available. Adrenaline and noradrenaline are very short acting and are best given by infusion, but can be given in small increment boluses and may be the only pressors available in low resource settings.

The practice of preloading the patient, i.e. the administration of IV fluid prior to giving regional anaesthesia, is controversial. If there is any evidence of dehydration or hypovolaemia, normal hydration should be achieved by suitable IV fluid replacement before administering the spinal anaesthetic. In the normovolaemic patient, it is recommended that the IV infusion is started before giving a spinal anaesthetic and possibly give up to 1000 ml of crystalloid. When there is a degree of urgency (and provided the mother is normovolaemic), do not delay for the preload.

7.3 **Positioning the mother**

Correct positioning of the mother is essential for successful spinal and epidural placement. Even the most accomplished operator will fail if the patient is badly positioned. The mother may find it difficult to get into a good position because of the enlarged uterus and find it hard to keep still during a contraction. Getting the mother to stay in a good position is helped by giving her a careful explanation before the start and by the presence of a well trained assistant. If an assistant is not available, it is important to help the mother into the correct position and identify the anatomy of her spine before getting scrubbed for the procedure and draping.

The fundamentals of a good position are a well flexed spine, which overcomes the natural lumbar lordosis and opens up the spaces between the vertebrae, and an untwisted back which helps the operator orientate the tip of the needle and keep it in the midline. There are two basic positions—sitting and on the side.

7.3.1 **Sitting position**
Many find this easier, particularly in the obese mother, as it is easier to identify the midline. The CSF pressure is also greater in this posi-

tion so appears more readily in the hub when using narrow gauge needles. The mother should sit on the side of the bed with her feet supported by a stool high enough that her knees are higher than her hips – this increases flexion of the back. The part of the bed on which she sits should be level, flat and even, to prevent her twisting. Ask her to hold a pillow in front of her chest, place her chin on her chest and relax her shoulders and slump down into the bed. Discourage her from leaning forward. Ask her if she feels her back is twisted – she may be aware of small degrees of twisting that are not obvious to the observer. An assistant or the mother's partner can help her maintain the good position. See Figure 7.1.

7.3.2 **Lateral position**

The mother lies on her side (usually the left) with her back close to and parallel to the side of the bed. She should draw her knees up in front of her abdomen as far as they will go and her chin should rest on her chest. Place a pillow or rolled up blanket under her head to straighten the spine and place another between her knees to prevent the pelvis from tilting. Ensure that the legs are drawn up evenly to prevent twisting of the spine. See Figure 7.2.

7.4 **Skin preparation**

It is important to position the patient properly and then feel and identify the bony landmarks before getting scrubbed up and sterilizing the patient's back. The skin should be sterilized with an alcohol or iodine based skin preparation. Chlorhexidine in alcohol is the best

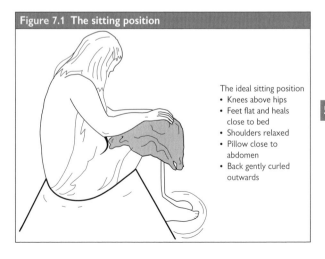

Figure 7.1 The sitting position

The ideal sitting position
- Knees above hips
- Feet flat and heals close to bed
- Shoulders relaxed
- Pillow close to abdomen
- Back gently curled outwards

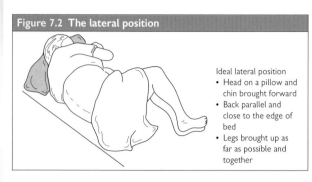

Figure 7.2 The lateral position

Ideal lateral position
• Head on a pillow and chin brought forward
• Back parallel and close to the edge of bed
• Legs brought up as far as possible and together

skin preparation. Double application with a gentle abrasive wipe and a sterile swab between applications is recommended. The final application should be allowed to dry naturally without wiping. An area at least 30 cm square should be prepared and drapes secured leaving only sterilized skin visible. If the operator has examined the back before hand, there should be no need to palpate bare skin further as this potentially brings to the surface viable bacteria from deeper skin layers.

7.5 **Technique of spinal needle insertion**

7.5.1 **Choice of needle**

The intrathecal (spinal) space is identified by the appearance of CSF in the hub of the spinal needle. Pencil point needles are better than Quincke designed needles as the incidence of headaches is greatly reduced. The diameter or bore of the needle also influences the incidence of post spinal headache. The lowest incidence is with 25 or 27 gauge needles but the operator should use the finest gauge with which he/she is familiar and can guarantee success. It is better to make a single puncture with a 22 gauge needle than try to use a finer needle but either fail or succeed only after several punctures of the dura. Spinal needles designed for single use should not be sterilized or re-used.

Where spinal needles are in short supply, it is possible to use the inner needle of a 20 gauge intravenous cannula as a substitute. These are sharper than true Quincke spinal needle and have a different 'feel' when traversing the tissue layers. The risk of headache is increased greatly with an IV cannula.

7.5.2 **Site of insertion**

The spinal cord ends at the level of the 1st lumbar vertebra but extends lower in some people. In order to avoid damage to the spinal cord, it is wise to insert the spinal needle no higher than between the 3rd and 4th lumbar interspace (L3/4) to avoid the possibility of spinal cord trauma. Truffier's line is the imaginary line between the two iliac crests and bisects the body of L4, hence the interspace immediately above this line is L3/4 and that immediately below is L4/5. See Figure 7.3.

Figure 7.3 Bony landmarks of the spine

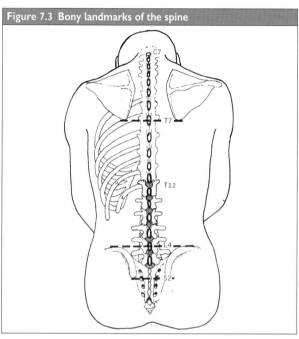

Figure 7.4 Subarachnoid and epidural spaces

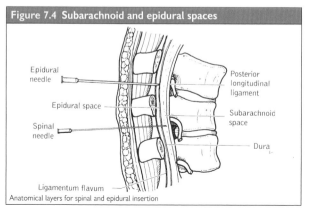

Epidural needle

Epidural space

Spinal needle

Posterior longitudinal ligament

Subarachnoid space

Dura

Ligamentum flavum

Anatomical layers for spinal and epidural insertion

Insertion sequence

1. Patient should have a patent IV line running.

2. Position patient (lateral or supine).

3. Identify and mark the relevant lumbar interspace (L3/4 or L4/5) and the midline.

4. Put on theatre hat and mask, scrub up and put on sterile gown and gloves.

5. Prepare skin as previously described.

6. Draw up intrathecal drugs ideally using a filter needle.

7. Infiltrate the skin with 25G needle using 2–5ml 1% lidocaine at and around the midpoint of the interspace.

8. Insert the introducer of the spinal needle until it is firmly gripped within the interspinous ligament.

9. Hold the spinal needle with the aperture usually directed cephalad and carefully introduce the spinal needle identifying the anatomical layers by 'feel' during insertion. See Figure 7.4.

10. A common problem is to hit bone before encountering the ligamentum flavum, in which case withdraw needle almost to skin and redirect needle and introducer upwards or downwards before advancing again.

11. Having identified the ligamentum flavum, push the needle forward a couple more millimetres until a gentle pop is felt.

12. Remove the stillette of the spinal needle and confirm placement by the appearance of CSF at the hub of the needle.

13. Stabilize the needle and syringe during injection with the back of the hand holding the needle braced against the mother's back.

14. It is usual to confirm CSF by gently aspirating on the syringe just before injection.

15. Re-confirming needle position by re-aspirating at the end of procedure is unnecessary as it is assessment of anaesthesia that will ultimately verify adequate injection.

16. Remove syringe, needle and introducer as one at the end of the injection.

7.6 **Choice of drugs for spinal anaesthesia**

A number of local anaesthetic drugs can be safely used and will depend on local availability. It is important that only sterile drugs are used and in a formulation that is not neurotoxic. Solutions may be normobaric (or slightly hypobaric), i.e. same density (or slightly less

Table 7.1 Suggested doses of local anaesthetic drugs			
Local anaesthetic	Concentration	Block for caesarean section	Duration of block
Bupivacaine (Plain or heavy)	0.5%	2–3 ml	2–3 hr
Lidocaine	2%	3–4 ml	30–45 min
Lidocaine	5%	1.2–1.6 ml	60–90 min
Cinchocaine (heavy)	0.5%	2–3 ml	2–3 hr
Tetracaine	1%	0.7–1.1 ml	2–3 hr
Tetracaine	0.5%	1.5–2.5	2–3 hr
Pethidine (meperidine)	50mg/ml	1.5 ml	

dense) than CSF or made hyperbaric i.e. denser than CSF by adding strong dextrose. Hyperbaric solutions will tend to sink in CSF and higher local anaesthetic concentrations will occur in dependant parts of the dural sac.

The dose should be reduced by around 40–50% when a perineal block is required eg perineal suturing

In addition to local anaesthetic drugs, it is possible to add other drugs which can slightly improve the quality of block or provide more prolonged postoperative pain relief. It should be stressed that it is not essential to use these adjuncts and their addition can increase the potential for drug error and complications. The most common class of adjunct drug is opiates. Short acting opiates, such as fentanyl (10–25mcg), may improve the quality of block while longer acting opiates, such as morphine (100 µg) and diamorphine (250mcg), can provide analgesia after the effect of local anaesthesia has worn off. However, the use of long acting opiates is associated with late respiratory depression (6–12 hr post op) and should only be used when there is adequate postoperative monitoring. It is essential that the formulation of opiate used is suitable for injection into the spinal space and is free of preservatives. Most morphine formulations contain preservative and are thus unsuitable.

7.7 Positioning the patient after insertion

It is important to reposition the mother as soon as the spinal injection has been made. Initially, she is placed flat on her back and then rapidly tilted to the left, either by using the operating tables lateral tilt facility to an angle of 15°, or by inserting a pillow, rolled up blanket or wedge under the right buttock to tilt the pelvis to around 15°. This will help to prevent, or at least reduce, the fall in blood pressure that the onset of spinal anaesthesia will cause. Similarly, it is essential to check the heart rate and blood pressure every 2–3 minutes until the baby is born. You should also ask the mother to tell you if she starts to feel faint or nauseous as this is usually a sign of decreased blood pressure. Hypotension should be promptly treated by increasing the IV infusion rate and administering a vasopressor drug (see above).

7.8 **Testing the block**

Before the start of surgery, it is important to ensure that the block is adequate for the operation. This can be done in a number of ways and relies on stimulating the mother on one side of her body, starting at the groin and first progressing towards the head until the mother says that sensation is normal. Different sensations can be used, such as temperature with ice or ethyl chloride, pin prick using a blunt needle, or light touch using cotton wool or a finger. Both sides should be tested as it is possible to have a denser block on one side. Next the lower extent of the block should be tested by stimulating from the groin down the leg to the sole of the foot. In contrast to an epidural, which can produce a band of anaesthesia, a spinal anaesthetic usually has an upper but no lower level to the block. Nonetheless, it is best to confirm this by checking down to the soles of the feet. An adequate block for caesarean section is one that reaches on both sides to the level of the lower part of the breast nipple (T4) to temperature and pin prick and to the level of the bottom of the rib cage near the midline or xyphisternum (T6) to touch. She should also have dense motor block of her legs and should be unable to perform a straight leg raise off the bed.

A useful confirmation of a good sensory block is to firmly pinch the patient just below the umbilicus. It is acceptable for her to feel some sensation but she should not detect it as a sharp pinch. See Figure 7.5.

7.9 **Problems with the block**

1. Block comes on slowly or is inadequate—depending on the drug used, spinal anaesthesia is usually achieved within 10 minutes but occasionally it may take longer. The block can be encouraged to spread upwards by bending the mother's knees up or tilting the operating table slightly head down. If not adequate within 20 minutes, another course of action is required. Complete failure can be managed by a repeat attempt if there is no urgency of delivery. A partial but inadequate block is more difficult to deal with. If there is time and the operator has the skills and resources, an epidural can be sited and the block brought up

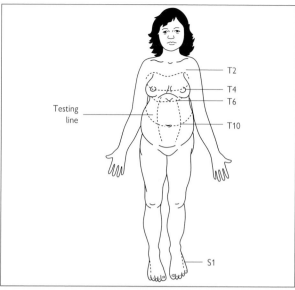

Figure 7.5 Sensory block for caesarean section. The sensory block should be tested 5cm from the midline. S1 should be blocked to all modalities. No sensation of pinching below T10. No sensation of light touch (rubbing ice cube) below T6. No sensation of cold below T4. Sensaton of icy cold at T2.

with epidural increments of local anaesthetic. More usually, it is better to proceed to general anaesthesia but remember that an incomplete block can still produce a degree of hypotension, which may be compounded by general anaesthesia

2. Hypotension— A greater than 20% fall from baseline or systolic pressure <90 requires treatment. Ensure that the patient is in a good position to reduce aortocaval compression (tilted 15° to left). Increase the IV infusion rate. Give bolus of vasopressor (see above for suggested drugs and doses) and repeat if blood pressure has not improved after 1 minute

3. Nausea and vomiting—usually a symptom of cerebral hypoperfusion and hypotension, so treat as 2. If BP confirmed as normal and still vomiting, consider giving an anti-emetic drug.

4. Pain during surgery—if pain is apparent, the mother must be reassured that it will be dealt with and the surgeon must be informed to stop. Depending on the stage of surgery and facilities available, IV opioids, IV ketamine, oxygen/N_2O may be administered, local anaesthesia infiltrated or a GA may be performed.

7.10 **Management after surgery**

After surgery, the mother is transferred to her bed and taken to a recovery or ward area. Although she is likely to be wide awake, in all other ways she should be treated the same as a woman who has had a caesarean section under general anaesthesia as she is liable to the same surgical complications. She will require regular observations of pulse, blood pressure and respiratory rate.

With regards to her recovery from the spinal anaesthetic, depending on the drug used, full motor power and sensation usually returns within 6 hours. It is important that she remains in bed at least until normal power and sensation has returned. Many institutions place a urinary catheter at the time of surgery and leave it in place for 12–24 hours after the operation. If a catheter is not left in place, the mother should be monitored closely for any signs of urinary retention (lower abdominal pain/discomfort and not passed urine).

7.11 **Spinal anaesthesia for other procedures**

Spinal anaesthesia can be used for other obstetric procedures such as perineal repair, evacuation of placenta and forceps delivery. See Chapter 19 for more detail.

- Perineal repair—usually a low spinal block involving just the sacral roots is required. In addition to a lower volume of local anaesthetic solution, spread can be restricted by using hyperbaric solution and keeping the patient sat up after spinal injection for 5 minutes
- Removal of retained placenta—requires a block of uterine innervation. Although the uterus is supplied by spinal segments T10–L1, to ensure a dense block of the uterus, it is best to aim to achieve a block to around T8
- Forceps delivery—requires just perineal and uterine anaesthesia suggesting a block to T8. However, if the surgeon wants the option to proceed straight to caesarean section if vaginal delivery fails, a high sensory block to T4 is required.

Chapter 8

Epidural anaesthesia

Rafal Baraz, Paul Clyburn

Key points

- Epidural anaesthesia is safe if inserted by a skilled practitioner where adequate monitoring and resuscitation can be provided
- Epidural anaesthesia requires good understanding of: the anatomy of the back and spine, physiological changes of pregnancy and the pharmacological effects of local anaesthetics
- Correct positioning of the mother is crucial to the success of epidural insertion
- It is very important to keep control of the epidural needle at all times during insertion
- Withdrawing the catheter through the epidural needle may shear the catheter. The catheter and needle should be removed as one unit
- Accidental dural puncture is an important complication
- Aspirating CSF through an epidural catheter is sometimes difficult and dural puncture by the catheter can be easily missed
- Test doses increase the safety of epidural anaesthesia and must be employed at all times
- Following accidental dural puncture, all top-ups must be given by an experienced anaesthetist.

8.1 Introduction

Epidural anaesthesia can be used to provide analgesia for labour pain. It requires identification of the epidural space (also called the extradural space) using a large calibre needle through which a catheter is inserted into the space. The incidence of complications associated with epidural anaesthesia is inversely proportional to the experience of the operator. Therefore, epidural analgesia in labour must be provided by a trained practitioner in a unit that is equipped with appropriate monitoring and adequate resuscitation facilities. The use of a catheter allows the maintenance of analgesia with further additional doses (top-ups) of local anesthetic solutions. An epidural that provides good quality analgesia for labour can also be used for caesarean section, forceps delivery, perineal suturing, and manual removal of placenta, by increasing the spread and density of block using appropriate concentrations and volumes of local anaesthetic solutions.

8.2 **Differences from spinal anaesthesia**

Although epidural anaesthesia, in many aspects, is similar to spinal anaesthesia, the two procedures are different and must not be confused with each other (see Table 8.1).

Table 8.1 Differences between spinal and epidural anaesthesia		
	Spinal anaesthesia	**Epidural anaesthesia**
Space	Subarachnoid space	Extradural space
Needle end point	Through dura and arachnoid (into CSF)	Between ligamentum Flavum and the dura
Needle size	Very small (22–27 gauge)	Large (16–19 gauge)
Insertion site	Only performed below L3	Can be performed at any spinal level
Mechanism of action	Spinal nerve roots and spinal cord	Spinal nerve roots
Local anaesthetic volume	Small volume (2–3 ml)	Large volume (15–30 ml)
Pharmacological effects	Immediate (5–10 min)	Delayed (10–30 min)
Side effects (e.g. hypotension)	Exaggerated	Moderate
Block density (motor block)	Very dense	Dense
Surgical conditions	Excellent	Very good
Extending the block	Not possible unless catheter technique	Catheter allows further top ups
Uses	Mainly for operative delivery	Labour analgesia and operative delivery
Cost	Inexpensive	Relatively expensive

8.3 Equipment

The basic equipment is the same as for spinal anaesthesia (see Chapter 7). In addition you will need:

- Sterile epidural pack containing epidural needle (Tuohy 16 or 18 gauge), loss of resistance syringe, epidural catheter and bacterial filter
- Saline 0.9%
- Sterile clear dressing over insertion site
- Dressing to secure catheter in place
- Epidural solution.

8.3.1 Epidural needle

The epidural needle is used to insert the catheter into the epidural space. The most commonly used is the Tuohy needle (16 or 18 gauge). The standard length is 8 cm with surface markings at 1cm intervals (a 11 cm extra long needle is also available). The overall length of the standard Tuohy needle is 10.5 cm. The tip is relatively blunt and slightly angled upward to encourage cranial direction of the catheter. Modern designs have detachable wings at the proximal end that allow more control of the needle during insertion. The needle has a stylet to prevent blockage with skin, fat, or ligament particles from the initial insertion.

8.3.2 Epidural catheter

The catheter is usually made of radio-opaque nylon with three lateral end holes all within 1.5 cm from its distal tip. Single end-hole catheters are less popular because they are associated with less effective blocks. The catheter usually has surface markings, which indicate how much catheter has been inserted: typically at 1 cm intervals between 5–15 cm with an overall length of 90 cm. Following insertion of the epidural catheter, the proximal end is attached to a dedicated bacterial filter through a connector. The catheter is inserted into the small lumen of the connector as far as it stops then twisted to secure. The primed epidural filter is then attached to the connector.

8.4 Procedure

8.4.1 Preparation and position

The mother is given a full explanation, positioned and the skin sterilized and the back draped as for spinal anaesthesia (see Chapter 7). It is recommended that the ideal inter-vertebral space for epidural insertion is palpated and marked prior to skin preparation, i.e. T12–L5 for labour analgesia.

8.4.2 **Epidural insertion**

Full aseptic conditions must be carried out throughout the procedure. Check and assemble the epidural kit. Flush the epidural catheter with saline to ensure patency and prime the epidural filter. The most popular way to identify the epidural space is by a loss of resistance technique, whereby constant finger pressure is maintained on the plunger of a syringe filled with saline attached to the Tuohy needle while advancing the needle. Air can be used instead of saline but requires a glass or non-sticking plastic syringe (See Figure 8.1a–c).

8.4.2.1 *Midline approach*

- Using 25G (25 mm) needle midway between the two identified spinous processes, infiltrate the skin and subcutaneous tissue with 3–5 ml of 1% lidocaine
- Infiltrate perpendicularly in the midline until the supraspinous ligament is encountered. This can be as superficial as 1 cm in the slim or as deep as 5 cm in the morbidly obese patient
- Insert Tuohy needle (with the stylet in place) through the skin, subcutaneous tissue and supraspinous ligament. The needle must remain in the midline at all times
- Once the supraspinous ligament is encountered with the epidural needle, remove the stylet and connect the loss of resistance syringe
- If using saline, apply constant pressure on the syringe plunger with one hand. Using the thumb and index finger of the other hand, hold the needle using its wings. The middle, ring and little fingers should be supported against patient's back to prevent any sudden movement of the needle during insertion (Figure 8.1a–c)
- Once the ligamentum flavum is encountered, resistance will increase further. Advance the needle very carefully by continuous pressure on the plunger until loss of resistance is obtained. Alternatively, advance the needle 1 mm at a time by holding the wings using the thumb and index finger of both hands and then checking for loss of resistance
- If using air, the thumb and index finger of both hands may be used to advance the needle 1 mm at a time and intermittently balloting the plunger until loss of resistance is achieved
- Once the epidural space is identified, minimal air or saline should be injected. Large volume of air may lead to a patchy block. Excessive volume of saline may confuse the identification of CSF
- Make a note of the depth of the epidural space from the skin
- Remove syringe from epidural needle and look for any clear fluid (CSF) or blood. It is not unusual to see a few drops of clear liquid coming out of the needle hub if saline is used

- The flow of saline drops usually slows down and eventually stops, while CSF continues to flow at a constant rate. If the dura is fully punctured with the needle, CSF will flow in excessive amount. If in doubt, check the exuded fluid for the presence of glucose

- The epidural catheter must be inserted very gently into the epidural space. Paraesthesia is common and the mother should be warned prior to insertion

- Paraesthesia is usually mild and transient. Excessive paraesthesia may warrant removal of the catheter with the needle and starting again

- Insert the catheter through the needle approximately 10cm in excess of the depth of the space from skin and then remove the needle

- When the needle is removed over the catheter, take care not to dislodge it: feed the catheter further as the needle is removed

- Once the needle is completely removed, pull the catheter out leaving 4 cm in the epidural space. Example: if the depth of the epidural space is 5cm from the skin, leave the catheter at 9 cm to skin

- Connect the small end of the special connector to the catheter. Screw the catheter firmly. If screwed very tightly, the connection may block the catheter itself

- Inject 0.5 ml of saline 0.9% through the catheter first and then aspirate with a 2 ml syringe and look for blood or CSF. Often, it is possible to aspirate clear fluid (up to 0.5 ml) from the catheter if saline was used. If more than 0.5 ml is aspirated, it should raise suspicion of an intrathecal catheter

- Lowering the proximal end of the catheter below the level of insertion will encourage passive flow of blood (if in an epidural vein) or CSF (if accidental intra-thecal placement). It is not uncommon to see clear fluid dripping from catheter end if saline is used. CSF usually flows at a constant rate while saline flow often slows down

- Secure the catheter in place. Ensure the catheter markings are clearly seen through a clear dressing. The rest of the catheter should be secured over the back and the shoulder.

8.4.2.2 *Paramedian approach*

If it is difficult to find the epidural space using a midline approach, a paramedian approach may be successful. The insertion point is one finger breadth (1–2 cm) from the midline at the level of the spinous process. Infiltrate with local anaesthetic first and then insert the epidural needle perpendicular to the skin until the lamina is encountered. Redirect the needle approximately 30° cephalad and 15° medially walking off the lamina. Once the ligamentum flavum is encountered, resistance to injection increases further, followed by sudden loss of resistance as the tip of the needle enters the epidural space.

Figure 8.1 Different hand hold techniques for epidural insertion. The left hand stabilizes the needle and the right hand places constant pressure on the plunger of the epidural syringe

(a)

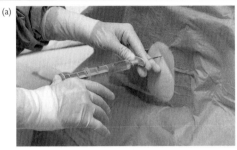

(b)

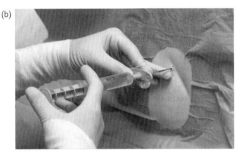

(c)

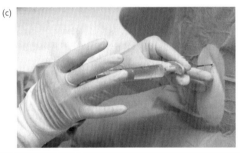

8.5 **Problems during insertion**

1. **Unable to locate epidural space**: usually the operator encounters bone in most directions. The two most common causes are suboptimal maternal positioning and failure of the operator to identify or remain in the midline during insertion. Check patient position. Ensure the spine is not twisted. The feet should be flat on a stool with the lower legs parallel to each other. Adopt a position that improves flexion of the spine by reducing lumbar lordosis. This can be achieved if the patient's knees are brought above the level of the hips. Also, lumbar lordosis can be reduced by tilting the bed 5 degrees towards the anaesthetist if this is possible. If still unsuccessful, attempt insertion in the lateral position or try the paramedian approach.

2. **Unable to thread the catheter**: most epidural packs contain a small catheter stabilizer, which attaches to the hub of the needle. This usually makes feeding the catheter easier. If unsuccessful, advance the epidural needle as little as 0.5 mm to ensure most of the needle bevel is within the epidural space or inject a few mls of saline to expand the epidural space. If still unsuccessful, re-do the epidural at a different level.

3. **CSF in the needle**: if the operator is familiar with the management of an intra-thecal catheter, feed the catheter into the intrathecal space, label it 'Spinal Catheter' and use with care, or re-site at a different site. Be aware of the risk of another dural puncture.

4. **Clear liquid in the needle**: It is not unusual to see a few drops of clear liquid coming out of the hub of the needle if saline is used for loss of resistance. The flow of saline drops usually slows down and eventually stops while CSF continues to flow. If in doubt, check for the presence of glucose in the fluid or feed the catheter and give a test dose.

5. **Blood tap**: this indicates that the needle or catheter had entered an epidural vessel. A tap with the needle requires re-siting. If there is blood in the catheter, withdraw the catheter leaving 3–4 cm length in the epidural space, flush with saline and aspirate again. If blood stops aspirating, lower the catheter tip below the insertion site and look for free flow of blood. If there is no blood, the catheter can be used cautiously. If blood continues to flow, resite the epidural at a different site.

6. **Pain during needle insertion**: if pain is experienced during needle insertion, identify the type and source of the pain. If the pain is localised to the back (soft tissue) then inject more local anaesthetic. If the needle is against the periosteum, then redirect the needle. If it is 'shooting' or 'electric shock' type of

pain (which suggests nerve irritation), stop advancing the needle, withdraw and then redirect the needle away from the side of the pain and continue. If pain recurs, try inserting at a different level.

7. **Pain on catheter insertion**: transient tingling sensation or a feel of an electric shock on catheter insertion is not unusual. However, persistent severe pain requires a re-site of the epidural.

8.6 Epidural for labour analgesia

8.6.1 Establishing the block

Once an epidural is inserted for labour, an appropriate block should be established. The possibility of intrathecal and intravascular placement cannot be ruled out until the epidural is tested. Following a test dose (see below), bolus doses of local anaesthetic solutions are injected to give sufficient analgesia. In the first stage of labour, this is usually achieved with a dermatone block of T10 to L1. For second stage pain, the block needs to be extended from T10 to S5. As the block for labour pain does not need to be as dense as for surgical procedures, low LA concentrations and doses are suitable.

8.6.2 The test dose

The test dose aims to detect intra-thecal and occasionally subdural placement of the catheter. The ideal test dose should be large enough to detect catheter misplacement but not too excessive to cause a total spinal or cardiovascular toxicity and collapse. A suitable example is bupivacaine 10mg (10 ml of 0.1% or 4 ml 0.25%).

8.6.2.1 Intravascular catheter

Early signs and symptoms of local anaesthetic toxicity can develop during injection of the test dose if the epidural catheter is in an epidural vessel. Warn and question the parturient about the possibility of numbness around the mouth, lightheadedness, tinnitus and confusion.

Table 8.1 Epidural doses			
Labour analgesia			
Local anaesthetic	Test dose	Initial dose	Top ups
Bupivacaine 0.1%	10 ml	10 ml + 10 ml	10 ml
Bupivacaine 0.25%	4 ml	5 ml + 5 ml	5 ml
Lidocaine 1%	5 ml	10 ml + 10 ml	10 ml
Surgical procedures			
Local anaesthetic	Dose		
Bupivacaine 0.5%	20 ml		
Lidocaine 2%	20 ml		

If in doubt, adrenaline (10–15mcg) can be injected down the epidural catheter to induce maternal tachycardia. If a diagnosis of an intravascular catheter is made, injection must be stopped and the catheter removed and inserted at a different level.

8.6.2.2 *Intrathecal catheter*

Following the administration of the initial test dose, signs that suggest/confirm intrathecal catheter placement are:

- Immediate labour analgesia (rapid drop in pain scores)
- Block higher than expected (possibly block to T6)
- Early motor block (unable to straight leg raise or knee flexion)
- Early sacral block (loss of ankle plantar flexion)
- Possibly hypotension.

8.6.2.3 *Management of intrathecal catheter*

Once an intrathecal catheter is identified:

- Place the woman in the left lateral position
- Give intravenous fluids and vasopressors to support the blood pressure if it falls
- Label the catheter clearly as 'Spinal Catheter'
- Inform the midwife and all members of the team
- Careful top-ups given by an experienced anaesthetist
- Ideal dosing for labour analgesia is one third of the dose of bupivacaine used for caesarean section given every 60–90 min, i.e. ~3–5mg of bupivacaine per top-up.

Chapter 9

Complications of regional anaesthesia

Paul Clyburn, Rafal Baraz

Key points

- A high regional block is more common than a total spinal, but it should be carefully observed as it may progress to a total spinal
- Total spinal is an emergency that requires immediate recognition and management (ABCD approach)
- Hypotension after spinal anaesthesia is common and should be treated by minimizing aorto-caval compression and vasopressors
- Prevention of local anaesthetic toxicity is easier than treatment
- Post dural puncture headache is common, it is typically postural in nature but should be differentiated from less common, more sinister causes of headache
- Epidural haematoma and abscess are uncommon but potentially very serious complications in which early recognition is important.

Although regional anaesthesia can reduce maternal morbidity and mortality, it is not without complications, even in the hands of experienced clinicians. As some complications are life threatening, early diagnosis and effective treatment is essential to ensure maternal and fetal wellbeing. Thus, the safe performance of regional anaesthesia requires the clinician to be able to recognize and manage these complications.

9.1 High block

A neuraxial block that has spread above the desired level intended for anaesthesia for caesarean section (T4 for cold) is called a high block. It may occur following: spinal anaesthesia alone, a large epidural top up or spinal anaesthesia that is given shortly after an epidural block.

The height of the spinal or epidural block is influenced by the dose of local anaesthetic injected, the patient's height and weight, patient position, and speed of spinal injection.

Hypotension due to increased sympathetic block is a prominent feature together with bradycardia resulting from blockade of cardio-accelerating fibres (T1–4). The patient may initially notice 'pins and needles' in the hands, followed by weakness in the upper limbs if the block extends to C5–T1 (brachial plexus). The patient may become quite anxious.

9.1.1 Treatment

Observe the patient closely as this may progress to a total spinal, place two pillows or a wedge under the shoulders to prevent further cranial spread of local anaesthetic, and give O2 via face mask and assess tidal volume. It is important to reassure the patient. If the patient is able to squeeze your hand and talk, she is able to maintain adequate ventilation. Bradycardia should be treated with anticholinergic drugs e.g. atropine 300–600mcg. Fluids and vasopressors are given to correct hypotension and aorto-caval compression is reduced by full left lateral position or left tilt with a pillow or wedge under the right hip.

9.2 Total spinal

Total spinal is life threatening and requires immediate recognition and management. It occurs when local anaesthetic spreads high into the cervical part of the spinal cord and the brain stem. Spread of LA above C5 blocks the phrenic nerve (C3, 4, 5) and the vasomotor center in the medulla oblongata leading to breathing difficulty, respiratory arrest, loss of consciousness and cardiovascular collapse.

Usually, it follows the injection of a large volume of high concentration local anaesthetic into the spinal or epidural space. It is more likely following epidural anaesthesia rather than single shot spinal owing to the larger volume used. It can occur when epidural local anaesthetic leaks into the spinal space through an unrecognized dural puncture (commonly after a difficult epidural insertion), or rarely when an epidural catheter migrates into the spinal space. This is only theoretically possible as it is difficult for the catheter to migrate through the tough dura; however, a misplaced subdural catheter can break the thinner arachnoid layer following injection of a large volume of LA. It can also occur when spinal anaesthesia is given shortly after an epidural top-up.

9.2.1 Clinical features

The features are a more extreme version of those in a high block but they progress more rapidly following injection of local anaesthetic, i.e. within a few minutes. The mother will quickly develop severe

> **Box 9.1 Treatment of total spinal**
>
> Immediate recognition and treatment is vital and should follow an ABC approach:
>
> **Airway**—Give high concentration oxygen and support the **airway**; if unconscious, apply cricoid pressure
>
> **Breathing**—Assist ventilation if apnoea develops and proceed with tracheal intubation. Use small doses of induction agent. Give ketamine or a reduced dose of thiopental (1/4 of normal dose) followed by suxamethonium
>
> **Circulation**—Check blood pressure, give fluids and vasopressors to treat hypotension (ephedrine 9–12mg increments) and atropine 300–600mcg to treat bradycardia; adrenaline 10–20mcg is effective in treating hypotension and bradycardia (larger doses are required in more severe cases)
>
> **Delivery** of the baby may be required. Discuss this with the obstetricians.
>
> If cardiac arrest develops, start cardiopulmonary resuscitation.
> Explain to the mother what has happened.

hypotension and bradycardia, nausea and vomiting, breathing difficulties, she becomes unable to speak followed by unconsciousness. Unless treatment is prompt, she will rapidly progress to cardiorespiratory arrest. See Box 9.1.

9.3 Hypotension

Hypotension is commonly defined as a drop of systolic blood pressure below 100 mmHg or a fall of more than 20% from baseline.

9.3.1 Physiological considerations

The degree of hypotension depends on the density and the extent of the sympathetic blockade. Hypotension is more evident after a spinal than an epidural blockade. Sympathetic block up to T5 will result in: dilatation of the resistance vessels (arteries) and consequently reduction in systemic vascular resistance; dilatation of the capacitance vessels (veins) leads to venous pooling and reduction in venous return; a reduction in endogenous catecholamine secretion from the adrenal medulla due to splanchnic nerve block; sympathetic block above T5 drops blood pressure further due to bradycardia; and reduction in myocardial contractility (nerve supply to myocardium T1–4).

9.3.1.1 Aortocaval compression

Also called supine hypotension and caused by occlusion of the inferior vena cava (IVC) and aorta by the gravid uterus when the mother is placed flat on her back. Occlusion of the IVC significantly reduces the venous return and as a result, the cardiac output. Occlusion of the aorta increases afterload and further reduces cardiac output.

Supine hypotension can occur as early as 20 weeks' gestation and becomes more obvious in the third trimester due to the increase in uterine size. Other risk factors are polyhydramnios, multiple pregnancy, maternal obesity, and uterine myomata.

Supine hypotension is less severe after membrane rupture, engagement of the fetal head and descent of the head through the pelvis and is unlikely to take place after delivery.

9.3.2 Minimizing the risk of hypotension

9.3.2.1 Prevent aortocaval compression

The aim is to displace the uterine plane from that of the aorta and inferior vena cava to minimize the compression. Place a wedge under the right hip to displace the uterus if the patient is still in the supine position. This requires twisting of the spine and is not ideal if the mother has pre-existing back problems. Uterine displacement is better performed by 15° left lateral tilt of the operating table. However, this does not reliably prevent aortocaval compression because of incomplete relief of vena cava compression. A more extreme 30° tilt or semilateral 45° position is more effective but not practical as the mother feels unsafe and surgical access is difficult.

The full lateral position is safe and most effective in avoiding aortocaval compression. When blood pressure is stable, the 15° left lateral tilt should be resumed and surgery may start.

9.3.2.2 Intravenous prehydration (preload)

Studies have consistently shown that hypotension cannot be eliminated even by a large crystalloid bolus before spinal anaesthesia.

Cystalloids have a short intravascular half-life. Therefore, if given, should be while spinal anaesthesia is instituted (called co-load).

A large crystalloid preload precipitates haemodilution and may cause the release of atrial natriuretic peptide (vasodilator), which may lead to persistent hypotension. Also, in pregnancy, the low colloid oncotic pressure can be decreased further by a large preload, potentially leading to pulmonary oedema.

Colloids are more effective in the prevention of hypotension as a result of slower redistribution out of the intravascular space leading to a more sustained increase in central venous pressure. This benefit must be weighed against their increased cost, lesser availability and the incidence of adverse reactions (allergic reactions, pruritus, and interference with blood cross-matching).

9.3.2.3 Lower limb wrapping

There is evidence to suggest that wrapping of the legs with tight elasticated bandages prior to spinal anaesthesia can reduce the incidence of hypotension.

9.3.3 **Treating hypotension**

Ephedrine and phenylephrine are the most widely used and studied vasopressors worldwide. They are used for both prophylaxis and treatment of hypotension. Atropine should be used to treat hypotension associated with bradycardia. Adrenaline can be given if other vasopressors are unavailable. It requires dilution to 10mcg/ml given in 1–2 ml boluses (1 ml 1:1000 adrenaline in 100 ml of saline, or 1 ml 1:10 000 adrenaline in 10 ml saline).

9.4 **Local anaesthetic (LA) toxicity**

Local anaesthetic toxicity is a potential complication when large amounts of LA drugs are used within a short period of time. Toxicity develops following the systemic absorption of local anaesthetic injected into the epidural space in excessive quantity. Toxicity after a smaller dose may develop if LA is inadvertently injected directly into an epidural blood vessel. In addition, deaths have been reported following unintentional LA injection directly into an IV cannula. Toxicity is unlikely during spinal anaesthesia as the volume used is very small.

Toxicity is directly proportional to LA drug potency (bupivacaine and ropivacaine are more toxic than lidocaine, prilocaine and mepivacaine).

9.4.1 **Prevention**

Detecting epidural vein cannulation may be difficult as excessive negative pressure may collapse the vein and mask intravascular placement. It is important to aspirate gently from the epidural catheter or hold the open end of the catheter below the level of the patient looking for blood coming back down the catheter. Always use a test dose when establishing an epidural block. Never exceed the safe recommended dose of LA and stop injecting if the woman develops early signs of toxicity.

9.4.2 **Signs and symptoms**

The presentation may vary depending on the concentration and the rate of rise of local anaesthetic in the plasma. As the brain is more sensitive to local anaesthetics, CNS manifestations tend to occur first followed by respiratory and cardiovascular manifestations. Convulsions may be the first signs if LA is injected rapidly and directly into a blood vessel.

Table 9.1 Signs and symptoms of local anaesthetic toxicity

CNS manifestations	CVS manifestations
• light-headedness	• hypotension and bradycardia
• tinnitus	• tachycardia and hypertension if LA
• circumoral numbness	contains adrenaline
• tongue paraesthesia	• arrhythmias
• blurred vision	• atrioventricular heart block
• drowsiness and confusion	• ventricular tachycardia (VT)
• loss of consciousness	• ventricular fibrillation (VF)
• convulsions	• asystole
• respiratory arrest	

9.4.3 Management

Early recognition of toxicity is vital. **STOP INJECTION.** The out-come depends on the extent of myocardial toxicity. An ABC approach is important:

- Give 100% oxygen
- Support the airway, if unconscious, apply cricoid pressure and intubate
- Assist ventilation if apnoea develops
- Check blood pressure, give fluids and vasopressors (ephedrine, methoxamine or phenylephrine) to treat hypotension and atropine to treat bradycardia
- Adrenaline 10-20mcg is effective in treating hypotension and bradycardia. Consider an adrenaline infusion
- Minimize aorto-caval compression by appropriate positioning
- If cardiac arrest, start cardiopulmonary resuscitation
- Early delivery if maternal cardiac arrest
- Lipid rescue with an intravenous infusion of 20% Intralipid 500 ml over 30 minutes has been effective in managing cardiac arrest from bupivacaine toxicity.

9.5 Postdural puncture headache

A postdural puncture headache (PDPH) can follow accidental dural puncture with an epidural needle or catheter, or intentional puncture during spinal anaesthesia. Dural puncture with a size 16 or 18 gauge epidural needle is more likely to cause the headache when compared to pencil-point, small gauge, atraumatic spinal needles. Large bore (18–20 gauge) Quinke needles have a high incidence (20–50%) of PDPH.

Headache can be explained by the development of intracranial hypotension following excessive CSF leak from the dural tear/hole. Intracranial hypotension leads to traction on the intracranial structures and compensatory cerebral vasodilatation leading to severe headache.

9.5.1 **Presentation**

Women usually complain of excruciating frontal or occipital headache within the first 48 hours following dural puncture. Headache is characteristically postural in nature (exacerbated by sitting up and relieved by lying down) and often associated with neck stiffness and back pain. Nausea, vomiting, tinnitus, vertigo, dizziness, visual disturbances, photophobia may also be present.

9.5.2 **Differential diagnosis**

Even when the history is convincing of PDPH, other causes must be considered as their impact if missed can be devastating. Important differential diagnoses include: intracranial space occupying lesion, subdural or subarachnoid haemorrhage, meningitis, cerebral sinus venous thrombosis, cerebral infarction, and pre-eclampsia. Migraine and non-specific headache are more benign causes.

9.5.3 **Treatment**

If untreated, a post-dural puncture headache should resolve within 7–14 days. Supportive therapy such as rehydration, analgesia i.e. regular paracetamol, non-steroidal anti-inflammatory drugs and an opioid may have a limited and temporary effect. Although caffeine and sumatriptan (an anti-migraine treatment) promote cerebral vasoconstriction, they have proven mostly ineffective. The most effective method of treatment is an epidural blood patch where 15–20 ml of patient's own blood is injected into the epidural space to seal the dural tear.

9.6 **Epidural or spinal haematoma**

The risk of an epidural or spinal haematoma is increased if a woman has a bleeding disorder or is anti-coagulated. A high index of suspicion is required to aid the diagnosis.

9.6.1 **Presentation**

Classically, an epidural or spinal haematoma presents with a prolonged effect of regional anaesthesia, back pain, a sensory deficit and motor weakness on both sides. There may be disturbance of bladder and bowel functions. Emergency surgery to evacuate the haematoma is required.

9.7 **Epidural or spinal abscess**

This is a rare but potentially devastating complication of regional anaesthesia. If left untreated, it can cause paraplegia and death. The risk increases if aseptic conditions are not followed. It classically presents 24–48 hours following epidural or spinal insertion but may be longer. A high index of suspicion is required to aid the diagnosis. *Staphylococcus aureus* is the most common organism.

9.7.1 **Presentation**

An epidural or spinal abscess classically presents with severe, deep seated back pain and local tenderness. The patient may have signs of systemic infection with fever and rigor, leucocytosis and an elevated CRP. There may be neurological signs such as a sensory deficit or lower limb weakness progressing to paraplegia.

Antibiotics alone have limited value and emergency surgery is usually necessary to minimize severe paraplegia.

Chapter 10

Other local anaesthetic techniques

Rafal Baraz, Paul Clyburn

Key points

- Caesarean delivery with local anaesthetic infiltration requires a skilled surgeon
- The total mass of local anaesthetic should not exceed the maximum recommended dose
- Using a long needle minimizes the number of skin injections
- This technique is mostly applicable in parts of the world with limited anaesthetic backup.

10.1 Local infiltration

The use of local anaesthetic infiltration for caesarean delivery is rarely used in developed countries due to availability of regional anaesthesia and the increased safety of general anaesthesia. However, it has been used as a safe alternative in situations where both regional and general anaesthesia are contraindicated or difficult to perform.

10.1.1 Indications

Caesarean sections can be performed under local anaesthetic infiltration when the patient is not suitable for either regional and general anaesthesia (e.g. severe kyphoscoliosis), where there has been failure of both regional and general anaesthesia, there is lack of anaesthetic expertise, or there is a lack of adequate anaesthetic equipment (spinal needles, anaesthetic machine, and gas supply).

10.1.2 Advantages

Local infiltration serves as an alternative option to anaesthesia after failed intubation and/or failed regional anaesthetic and can also avoid the need for general anaesthesia and its complications (hypoxia, aspiration, awareness). It avoids haemodynamic changes that are associated with regional and general anaesthesia. In addition, blood loss is reduced as adrenaline is added to local anaesthetic (LA) and the surgeon can administer the anaesthetic and perform the caesarean.

10.1.3 **Disadvantages**

The technique is time consuming and requires multiple injections leading to increased discomfort. It is sometimes associated with a degree of pain and there is a risk of LA toxicity for the mother and the baby. There is also a risk of uterine perforation.

10.1.4 **Procedure**

Both the obstetrician and the mother must be prepared. The patient must be warned that some painful sensation as well as touch and pressure may be experienced. Drugs and equipment for resuscitation must be available prior to commencing the procedure. Ideally, an anaesthetist should be present to aid analgesia with Entonox or other analgesics if required.

10.1.4.1 *Technique*

Standard basic monitoring, large IV access and fluid infusion are a prerequisite and the procedure should be performed with the patient in the left lateral tilt position until the baby is delivered.

Suggested LA preparation—use 7mg/kg of either lidocaine or prilocaine 0.5–1% with 5mcg/ml adrenaline (1:200,000). A 100–120 mm needle is used to infiltrate under the skin. For the Pfannensteil incision, infiltrate LA along the incision line. For a vertical incision, local field block of the lower abdominal wall with multiple injections is required. It is more time consuming and associated with an increased degree of discomfort. LA is infiltrated from the umbilicus down to the symphysis pubis in the midline and 4 cm lateral to the midline. The abdominal wall, during pregnancy, may become very thin. Therefore, the needle should be kept under the skin to avoid uterine perforation. Once the skin is incised, the rectus sheath is infiltrated. The fat has minimal nerve endings, therefore infiltration with LA is not necessary and would waste a large volumes of LA. The parietal peritoneum is anaesthetized by injecting 10 ml of LA under the linea alba. Once the parietal peritoneum is opened, spray 10 ml of LA into the peritoneal cavity. Finally infiltrate 5–7 ml of LA into the visceral peritoneum of the lower segment of the uterus. This also helps to separate the peritoneum from the lower segment. Before delivery of the head, warn the mother about the risk of experiencing pain, especially if the head is engaged. Further injection of LA may be required during closure.

If supplementation with narcotic analgesics is required, it is best given after delivery of the baby. This technique is not perfect but it is of great value in providing anaesthesia for caesarean section, especially in countries with limited resources.

Chapter 11

Post delivery

Rafal Baraz, Paul Clyburn

> **Key points**
> - Post delivery monitoring reduces the incidence of maternal morbidity and mortality
> - All women who receive obstetric anaesthesia or analgesia should be reviewed by the anaesthetic team after delivery
> - Any delay in epidural or spinal block regression should be referred early to the anaesthetic team
> - Management of pain after delivery requires a multimodal approach
> - Withholding oral fluids after uncomplicated caesarean section has no benefit.

11.1 Monitoring and observations— what to look for

All women should be observed and monitored following delivery of the baby. The intensity of observations depends not only on the type of delivery but also on the anaesthetic and surgical intervention. Women with uncomplicated vaginal delivery often require minimal monitoring after delivery in contrast to those having emergency caesarean section or post partum haemorrhage.

All women who receive anaesthesia or regional labour analgesia should be reviewed by the anaesthetic team sometime between 18–36 hours after delivery. During the review, enquiries should be made about the effectiveness of the anaesthetic intervention and maternal satisfaction, whether there is any anaesthetic related morbidity, e.g. headache (associated with a post dural tap), nausea and vomiting, backache and whether the mother has adequate pain control. It is also important to confirm that the mother has made a full neurological recovery after regional anaesthesia, is mobilizing and able to pass urine. It is useful to review that her vital signs are normal and have been charted as required. Appropriate action should be taken when abnormal recordings are found.

11.1.1 **Observation charts**

Basic observations include monitoring of the vital signs, i.e. heart rate, blood pressure, respiratory rate, temperature, and where available pulse oximetry, sedation scores, and pain scores. These observations are required for all women. Uncomplicated vaginal delivery, with or without labour analgesia, should be monitored for the first few hours after delivery and then 12 hourly until discharge, but women delivered by caesarean section require closer observations. In the immediate postoperative period, observations should be performed every 15 minutes. Observations should be continued until full recovery from general anaesthesia is obtained. Monitoring every 2 hours is then required for the first 24 hours. Deliveries that are complicated with large blood loss or severe pre-eclampsia may need hourly observations for 24 hours or until their condition is stable with additional observation such as oxygen requirements, blood gases, blood count, urea and electrolytes, urine output, and fluid balance. A higher level of care may be needed if the patients' condition deteriorates. Women receiving long acting intrathecal/epidural opioids (morphine and diamorphine) and patient controlled analgesia (PCA) are at increased risk of respiratory depression and their observations must be performed every two hours for 24 hours. The coloured early warning observation chart (Chapter 15, Figure 15.1) has been introduced in some countries as a track and trigger tool. This is to help nurses and midwifery staff to identify sick women during the antenatal and postnatal periods. Early identification of these women then requires a timely response from the medical or surgical team before significant deterioration occurs.

11.1.2 **Block regression**

Block regression after spinal anaesthesia starts one hour following the injection of the standard surgical dose of bupivacaine. Larger doses may prolong the block. Epidural block, however, starts to regress approximately 2 hours following bupivacaine 0.5%. Most neuraxial blocks wear off completely after 12 hours and women are able to mobilize. However, if repeated doses of long acting local anaesthetic (such as bupivacaine) are used, full neurological recovery may be delayed up to 24 hours. Women should be observed closely following spinal and epidural blocks and any delay in neurological recovery should be referred to the anaesthetic team.

The block regresses in the following order: motor nerves recover first, then sensory and finally the autonomic nerves, with bladder sensation recovering last. All women should be reviewed at 24 hours to ensure full neurological recovery and women must not attempt to walk until motor block has recovered. When a woman is mobilizing for the first time, this should be aided by a nurse, midwife, or relative.

11.1.3 **Micturition**

Bladder sensation is the last function to recover following neuraxial blockade. The ability to micturate is especially prolonged if spinal or epidural opioids are administered. An indwelling urinary catheter is required for at least 12 hours to reduce the risk of bladder wall damage due to urine retention.

After the urinary catheter is removed, the women's ability to pass urine should be monitored. She should be encouraged to drink in order to maximize urine production and if after 6 hours the woman has not passed urine, it is important to determine whether this is due to urine retention or simply because of dehydration. The bladder should be palpated or an ultrasound scan performed, if available, to determine bladder volume. If there is evidence of urine retention, the bladder must be re-catheterized.

11.1.4 **Headache**

It is very important to differentiate post dural puncture headache from other types of headaches. Post dural puncture headache is usually severe, postural in nature and often associated with evidence of dural puncture with the epidural needle or multiple attempts at spinal anaesthesia (see Chapter 9).

11.1.5 **Backache**

Back pain is a very common symptom after delivery. Back pain during pregnancy may extend into the postnatal period and may take several weeks to resolve. New backache may develop after regional anaesthesia either as a localized or more generalized ache. Localized tenderness is common at the site of needle insertion and is related to local soft tissue haematoma. More generalized back pain may be due to musculoskeletal spasm. The mother should be reassured that this back pain is common and should resolve within a few days. Women should also be reassured that spinal or epidural anaesthesia is not associated with long-term back problems.

Although rare, if back pain is associated with other symptoms suggestive of epidural haematoma or abscess, urgent radiological examination and a neurosurgical opinion will be required.

11.1.6 **Nausea and vomiting**

There are many reasons why a mother may have nausea and vomiting after delivery, particularly if she had a caesarean section. Hypotension following regional anaesthesia, opioid use, antibiotic prophylaxis, and uterotonic infusions may all contribute to her symptoms. Occassionally, an ileus develops after delivery, especially after caesarean section. Persistent vomiting with abdominal distension should be managed with IV fluids, IV anti-emetics, and kept nil by mouth until the abdomen is soft.

11.1.7 **Fluid management and feeding**

Postoperative fluid administration aims to ensure adequate intravascular volume to maintain optimal organ perfusion. Postoperative fluid management should take into account the pre-operative deficit, blood loss during delivery and daily maintenance requirements.

Hypovolemia and dehydration following delivery may not only lead to maternal fatigue but could precipitate renal failure. Fluid overload, on the other hand, can be harmful as increased lung water leads to pulmonary oedema and increases the risk of pneumonia. Fluid overload also reduces gastric emptying and prolongs post-operative ileus.

If blood loss is more than 1000 ml, an intravenous fluid infusion should be started to replace the blood loss in addition to early oral intake. There is no evidence of benefit from withholding oral fluids after uncomplicated caesarean section. The incidence of nausea and vomiting is not increased by early fluid intake. Complicated caesarean sections (e.g. massive haemorrhage) may require further anaesthesia and therefore the patient should not be fed orally until reviewed by an obstetrician. Early oral fluid intake is associated with earlier first food intake, earlier return of bowel sounds and function and reduced abdominal distension. Women should therefore be encouraged to drink immediately following normal delivery and caesarean section and eat whenever they feel hungry.

11.2 **Pain control**

The severity of pain post delivery does not only depend on the mode of delivery but also on the type of anaesthetic used if any. It is best to use a multimodal approach (combination of paracetamol, NSAIDs and opioids) as this improves the efficacy of analgesia and allows reduced doses of individual agents.

11.2.1 **Vaginal delivery**

Pain after vaginal delivery is minimal, unless associated with an episiotomy or perineal tear. Regular paracetamol (1g 6 hourly) and NSAID (diclofenac 50mg 8 hourly or Ibuprofen 400mg 8 hourly) should provide adequate analgesia. More severe pain (3rd and 4th degree tears) can be controlled by adding codeine phosphate (60mg 6 hourly) or tramadol (50–100mg every 4–6 hours).

11.2.2 **Caesarean section**

11.2.2.1 *After regional anaesthesia*

The effect of morphine (100mcg intrathecally or 4mg epidurally) can last up to 18–24 hours and that of diamorphine (250mcg intrathecally or 5mg epidurally) can last up to 8–12 hours. If long-acting spinal opioids are used, further systemic opioids should be avoided in the first 12–24 hours following delivery. Oral or intravenous tramadol or codeine can be used during this period for breakthrough pain.

The combination of paracetamol and NSAID (if not contraindicated) is very efficacious and should be given immediately after caesarean delivery and on a regular basis.

11.2.2.2 *After general anaesthesia*

Caesarean sections performed under general anaesthesia often require intra-operative morphine, IV/PR paracetamol, IV/PR diclofenac and wound infiltration with local anaesthetic. Ideally, morphine PCA should be prescribed for postoperative pain, but a good alternative is IM morphine (10mg up to every 2 hours). Bilateral ilioinguinal nerve block or transverse abdominis plane block (performed before waking the woman up) are associated with lower pain scores and also reduce morphine requirement post delivery.

11.2.3 **Pharmacology**

11.2.3.1 *Paracetamol*

Paracetamol is a very safe drug during and after pregnancy and delivery. The dose is 1 g orally 4–6 hourly (maximum 4 g/24 hours). It is safe in therapeutic doses for women who are breast-feeding. An adjustment in dose is recommended in severe liver insufficiency.

11.2.3.2 *Non steroidal anti inflammatory drugs (NSAIDs)*

NSAIDs are very effective especially in combination with paracetamol, local anaesthetic blocks, and opioids. Diclofenac (oral, rectal, and IV) is the most commonly used agent and ibuprofen is a useful alternative. The suppository form is easy to administer and ideal in women suffering nausea and vomiting. It should be given at the end of the caesarean section if not contra-indicated. The IV form is ideal for caesarean section under general anaesthesia and after delivery of the baby. Usual doses are diclofenac 50–75mg PO/PR 8–12 hourly to a maximum of 150mg in 24 hours. It is safe in therapeutic doses for women who are breast-feeding. NSAIDs are contra-indicated in renal impairment, severe pre-eclampsia and major haemorrhage and are best avoided in women with history of peptic ulceration. If administered in therapeutic doses in the third trimester of pregnancy, NSAIDs can lead to premature closure of patent ductus arteriosus in the neonate and should not be given.

11.2.3.3 *Opioids*

Opioids are not routinely prescribed after vaginal delivery, but women who deliver by caesarean section under regional anaesthesia may receive intrathecal or epidural opioids to cover the postoperative period and are less likely to require additional opioids. After caesarean section under general anaesthesia, regular postoperative opioids are often required. Depending on availability and the local unit protocol, opioids can be given orally, intramuscularly (IM) or intravenously (IV). Oral morphine preparations are very effective and widely available. The oral route may not be ideal if the woman is experiencing nausea and vomiting, while the IM route is painful and requires administration by a nurse or midwife. Women should be monitored closely for 24 hours after intrathecal opioids and while receiving intravenous opioids. Naloxone should be prescribed and available on the maternity ward, and staff should be trained to use it if the mother's respiratory rate falls below 8 breaths/min.

11.2.3.4 *Patient controlled intravenous analgesia (PCIA)*
PCIA is an excellent method of pain relief especially after general anaesthesia for caesarean section. It is more effective than the oral or IM route and is associated with higher maternal satisfaction. Morphine is preferred over fentanyl because of its longer duration of action and over pethidine because of its minimal neonatal effects. Norpethidine is the active metabolite of pethidine and it accumulates in both the mother and the breastfed infant. Newborn babies exposed to pethidine may have impaired behaviour, increased risk of respiratory depression and seizures. A common dose for PCIA morphine is 1mg bolus with a lock out period of 5 minutes.

11.2.3.5 *Local anaesthetic blocks*
Wound infiltration with local anaesthetics provides excellent analgesia after caesarean section especially those performed under general anaesthetic. Bilateral ilioinguinal, iliohypogastic, and subcostal nerve blocks provide postoperative analgesia for caesarean section by blocking somatosensory fibres of T12 and L1. Bilateral transversus abdominis plane (TAP) blocks are also very effective. Local anaesthetic blocks can be performed at the end of the caesarean delivery or in the postoperative period. These blocks are more effective when combined with administration of NSAIDs and paracetamol.

11.2.3.6 *Postoperative epidural analgesia*
This can be employed for women who deliver by caesarean section under epidural or combined spinal-epidural technique. Although it is usual for an epidural catheter to be removed at the end of the caesarean delivery, this method of postoperative analgesia may be usefully employed in selected cases (e.g. women who may be allergic to morphine).

This can be used either as continuous infusion or as patient controlled epidural analgesia (PCEA). The same low dose solution used for labour analgesia can be used for postoperative analgesia.

Chapter 12

General anaesthesia

Stephen Morris, Eugène Zoumenou

Key points

- Obstetric anaesthetic practitioners need a safe, practised technique, which they can use with the resources available
- Thorough pre-operative assessment is essential
- Tracheal intubation helps protect against aspiration
- Correct positioning for intubation and uterine displacement is essential
- Extubation should be delayed until the mother is awake, breathing normally and has protective airway reflexes.

12.1 Introduction

Despite the increase of regional anaesthesia in obstetrics, general anaesthesia will always be necessary in cases where regional anaesthesia is contraindicated, refused, unavailable, or unsuccessful. The principles of general anaesthesia for caesarean section are to provide a well-oxygenated mother at a level of surgical anaesthesia with good perfusion of her brain and uterus whilst minimizing the risks of aspiration of gastric contents and awareness. This is a description of an ideal general anaesthetic technique for an emergency caesarean section, which may need to be modified where resources are limited.

12.2 Preoperative assessment

Even in the most urgent of cases, some form of pre-operative assessment must be carried out. The pre-operative evaluation will include a medical history to identify any relevant co-morbidities, a personal or family history of problems with general anaesthesia (including death or unexpected admission to intensive care or prolonged stay in hospital), any allergies and concurrent medication. Establish when the last solid and fluid intake was and where possible, explain to the mother what is going to happen and give her the opportunity to ask questions.

Assessment of the airway and prediction of difficult intubation are covered in Chapter 13.

An examination of the cardiovascular and respiratory systems should be done. It might be necessary to start fluid resuscitation prior to anaesthesia if there are any signs of shock: tachycardia, hypotension, cold extremities, tachypnoea, oliguria.

Take blood for a haemoglobin estimation and blood group and antibody screen where facilities exist. It is not necessary to wait for the result of the haemoglobin, but it may help guide peri-operative fluid and blood replacement in the event of haemorrhage.

12.3 **Anaesthetic technique**

Secure intravenous access with a 14–16g cannula and give 30 ml of 0.3 Molar sodium citrate (or other non-particulate antacid) orally and 50mg ranitidine intravenously. Check the anaesthesia machine, equipment, and prepare drugs (see Boxes 12.1 and 12.2).

Box 12.1 Equipment

Oxygen supply	Stethoscope
Anaesthetic circuit/face mask	Laryngoscope
Vaporizer	Bougie
Ventilator/Self-inflating bag	Tracheal tube size 7.0 mm
Suction apparatus	Tape
Tilting table	Syringe
Wedge/pillow	Laryngeal mask airway
Monitoring—ECG, NIBP, pulse oximeter, capnograph	Cricothyroid puncture device

---

Box 12.2 Drugs

Thiopental/(ketamine)
Suxamethonium
Non-depolarizing relaxant
Volatile agent
Oxytocin
Atropine

Analgesics—
- Fentanyl
- Morphine
- Paracetamol

Vasopressors—
- Ephedrine
- Phenylephrine

Position the patient supine with a pillow under their head and either tilt the table 15° to the left or place a support (e.g. a pillow or a rolled blanket) under the right hip to displace the uterus and minimise aorto-caval compression. Start monitoring with ECG, non-invasive blood pressure (NIBP), and pulse oximetry, and place the sucker under the pillow for rapid access.

Pre-oxygenate the patient for 3 minutes using a tight-fitting face mask and an oxygen flow rate of at least 10 L/min. It is important to remove as much nitrogen from the functional residual capacity (FRC) as possible, since this will act as a store of oxygen and prolong the time before hypoxia occurs if there is any difficulty in tracheal intubation. If the mother removes the mask and breathes room air, the pre-oxygenation time must start again.

Induction of anaesthesia is classically performed with a 'rapid sequence induction' technique. An assistant should perform cricoid pressure (Sellick's manoeuvre) to reduce the risk of regurgitation of gastric contents. Start with 10 Newton of force whilst the patient is awake (10 N is equivalent to a weight of 1 kg and can be practiced by pressing down on a weighing scales to the equivalent weight). Give 5mg/kg of sodium thiopental intravenously, and as soon as consciousness is lost, increase the force on the cricoid cartilage to 30 N and give 1.5mg/kg suxamethonium into a fast running intravenous infusion to avoid precipitation with the thiopental. Keep the face mask in place until the muscle fasciculation has finished and then intubate the trachea. If no fasciculation is seen, wait until 45 seconds have passed since injection of the suxamethonium and attempt intubation (for difficult intubation see Chapter 13). Inflate the cuff of the tracheal tube, secure it in place with tape or a tie, and ventilate the lungs. If a capnograph is available, the presence of carbon dioxide will confirm tracheal intubation. Check that air entry is present and equal on both sides by listening with a stethoscope over both lung apices or in the axillae. If the tube is passed too far into the trachea, it usually enters the right main bronchus and air entry will be diminished in the left apex. Once tracheal intubation has been confirmed, and the tube has been secured, the cricoid pressure can be removed. Make a note of how far in the correctly positioned tube has been inserted, as this will help detect movement of the tracheal tube during surgery. Manually check the pressure in the pilot balloon of the cuff to ensure it is not overinflated: 1ml of air after the leak has disappeared is sufficient. Ventilate the lungs with 50% oxygen in nitrous oxide (if available) and add 0.5–0.8 MAC of a volatile agent (e.g. 0.5% halothane or 1.0% isoflurane). Low concentrations of volatile agents (less than 1 MAC) do not increase bleeding by reducing uterine tone but will significantly reduce the incidence of awareness. Ventilate the lungs to an end-tidal carbon dioxide of 4.0%/4.0kPa, or at a tidal volume of 7 ml/kg and a frequency of 12–14 breaths/min. Heart rate, blood pressure and oxygen saturation should be recorded every 5 minutes.

After delivery of the baby, give 5 IU of oxytocin by slow intravenous injection. This can be repeated if necessary. Rapid injection of oxytocin in a hypovolaemic mother can cause severe hypotension. Intramuscular oxytocin 5 IU with ergometrine 250mcg (Syntometrine®) is an alternative. Antibiotic prophylaxis (e.g. co-amoxiclav 1.2g) against wound infection or endometritis can be given after clamping of the umbilical cord.

If the mother starts to breathe after the suxamethonium has worn off, a small dose of a non-depolarizing muscle relaxant, such as atracurium 0.2–0.3mg/kg, can be given if the respiratory effort is interfering with the surgery. After delivery of the baby, muscle relaxation is not essential for the surgery, but ventilation will need to be controlled until full return of muscle power.

Intravenous paracetamol 1g and morphine 10mg in divided doses should be given for postoperative analgesia.

At the end of the procedure, perform deep pharyngeal suction under direct vision with the help of a laryngoscope (never blindly), place a Guedel airway and administer 100% oxygen. Turn off the vaporizer but continue to ventilate the lungs to wash out the volatile agent. Place the mother in the left lateral position and slightly head-down. If a non-depolarizing muscle relaxant has been used, reverse the effects with neostgmine 2.5mg and atropine 1.2mg. Only extubate the trachea when the mother has regained consciousness and has demonstrated adequate return of muscle power. If a nerve stimulator is not available, power can be assessed clinically by the ability to lift the head off the bed for 5 seconds, protrude the tongue and squeeze the anaesthetist's hand. Extubation before the return of adequate muscle power will put the mother at risk of aspiration of gastric contents, and hypoxia/hypercarbia secondary to impaired respiratory function. The diaphragm is one of the first muscles to recover from neuromuscular blockade, but the beginning of respiratory effort does not mean there is adequate return of muscle power, especially in the pharyngeal and accessory muscles of ventilation.

12.4 Modifications

12.4.1 Hypertension

Induction of anaesthesia should be modified in the presence of hypertensive diseases of pregnancy to avoid the hypertensive response to laryngoscopy and intubation. Options include: intravenous lidocaine 1.5mg/kg, alfentanil 10–20mcg/kg, fentanyl 1–2mcg/kg, or magnesium sulphate 1–2g prior to the thiopental. If an opioid is used, there is a risk of neonatal respiratory depression requiring naloxone after delivery, so it is best avoided if the expertise to treat the newborn is not available.

12.4.2 **Magnesium sulphate**

If patients with pre-eclampsia or eclampsia are being treated with magnesium, the dose of non-depolarizing relaxant must be reduced by 50%. Magnesium reduces acetylcholine release at the neuromuscular junction and potentiates the effect of non-depolarizing muscle relaxants.

12.4.3 **Patient position**

Pillows may not be readily available, but it is nevertheless important to position something under the occiput to provide some neck flexion; a folded towel, a piece of material or even the patient's clothes can be used. Similarly, if the operating table does not tilt laterally, some displacement of the uterus can be achieved by placing some support (see above) under the patient's right buttock. Manual displacement of the uterus is equally, if not more, effective.

12.4.4 **Monitoring**

In the absence of ECG and pulse oximetry, monitoring will consist of manual palpation of a peripheral pulse and non-invasive blood pressure recordings. During induction and tracheal intubation, it is useful for somebody to monitor the patient's pulse for the anaesthetist. Adequacy of chest expansion and the colour of the mucous membranes should be assessed regularly.

12.4.5 **Oxygen concentrator/draw-over**

A draw-over system consists of a carrier gas, usually air with or without supplemental oxygen, which passes through a low-resistance vaporiser to a self-inflating bag or bellows and then on to the patient through a non-return valve. The system is robust and simple to understand and maintain.

In circumstances where the oxygen supply comes from an oxygen concentrator, the optimum pre-oxygenation seems to be a flow rate of 4 L/min for 3 minutes. Following intubation, ventilate the lungs with a self-inflating bag and non-return valve. Volatile anaesthetic agents can be added through a low resistance draw-over vaporizer (EMO/Oxford/triservice).

12.4.6 **Ketamine techniques**

Ketamine is an extremely useful drug that provides hypnosis, analgesia, and amnesia and is also a bronchodilator. If anaesthesia is induced slowly, the patient usually maintains their airway well. It can be used in a variety of techniques: by the intramuscular or intravenous route, by intermittent injection or continuous infusion, with or without tracheal intubation and controlled ventilation. However, general anaesthesia in the peripartum period without tracheal intubation is hazardous and should only be performed if absolutely necessary. Ketamine is relatively contra-indicated in patients with hypertension or pre-eclampsia because it causes an increase in blood pressure and intracranial pressure. However, this sympathetic stimulation is useful if patients are hypotensive or shocked. The other undesirable side-effects of salivation and postoperative hallucinations can be minimized by the use of atropine and diazepam. It is available in three concentrations, 10, 50, and 100mg/ml, for intramuscular use or it can be diluted for intravenous use. Because all women presenting for caesarean section will have venous access, the intramuscular route will not be discussed.

12.4.7 **Intermittent injection and spontaneous ventilation**

Induce anaesthesia with slow intravenous injection of 1–2mg/kg ketamine and 600mcg atropine. This will provide surgical anaesthesia for about 15 minutes. Maintain anaesthesia with intravenous injections of 0.5mg/kg ketamine according to the patient's response. Give oxygen by face mask or nasal cannulae and apply chin-lift and jaw thrust to maintain a clear airway. After delivery, give 0.1mg/kg intravenous diazepam.

12.4.8 **Intravenous infusion**

Dilute 500mg ketamine in 500 ml of Normal saline or Hartmann's solution to produce a 1mg/ml mixture. A standard intravenous giving set provides 20 drops/ml (you can confirm the drop size of your set by dripping fluid into the occluded barrel of a 2 ml syringe and counting the number of drops in 1 ml) so each drop contains 50mcg ketamine. If the infusion is used for induction of anaesthesia, a volume of 50–100 ml will be required for surgical anaesthesia. Test the depth of anaesthesia by pinching the patient's skin with forceps before skin incision.

For the maintenance of anaesthesia, an infusion rate of 1 drop per second is equivalent to 3mg/minute (60 drops per minute @ 50mcg per drop = 3,000mcg/min). The usual maintenance dose is between 1–5mg per minute, so the drop rate will need to be adjusted to between 1 drop every 3 seconds and approximately 5 drops every 3 seconds. Increased muscle tone with spontaneous movement of the limbs is sometimes seen.

Although ketamine provides intraoperative analgesia, intravenous opioids may still be required for postoperative analgesia. Intravenous morphine can be titrated after delivery and will reduce the intraoperative ketamine requirements but will also increase the risk of respiratory depression.

12.4.9 Unavailability of suxamethonium

If suxamethonium is unavailable, tracheal intubation can be facilitated with a non-depolarizing agent. Ideally this should be an agent with a relatively short duration of action, such as atracurium (in a dose of 0.5mg/kg) or vecuronium (0.1mg/kg), or a rapid onset of action, such as rocuronium (0.6mg/kg). The obvious disadvantage of these drugs is that they cannot readily be reversed in the event of difficulty with intubation and oxygenation. Unfortunately, in some countries, the only drug available may be pancuronium, which requires a modification of the induction technique. Pancuronium has a slow onset of action and a long duration of action. When used in a dose of 0.07mg/kg (approximately 4mg), it takes 3 minutes for a neuromuscular block of 90%, by which time the majority of the oxygen in the FRC will have been metabolized and hypoxia will occur very rapidly. The onset of action can be shortened to one minute by 'priming' with a small dose, one tenth of the total dose, 3 minutes before the main dose. The induction of anaesthesia would be as follows: start pre-oxygenation, give 0.5mg pancuronium, wait 3 minutes, give thiopental and remainder of pancuronium (3.5mg), wait one minute and then intubate the trachea. The duration of action of pancuronium with this technique is approximately one hour, so adequate time for recovery of muscle power must be allowed. This technique should *not* be used in patients receiving magnesium sulphate because of the exaggerated effect of the muscle relaxant in the presence of magnesium.

12.5 Summary

The main risks of general anaesthesia, namely airway complications resulting in failed intubation and aspiration of gastric contents can be avoided by the use of regional anaesthesia. The safe principles outlined above can be applied to any general anaesthetic in pregnancy and precautions against aspiration should be taken from the second trimester until 48 hours after delivery.

Chapter 13

Complications of general anaesthesia

Stephen Morris, Eugène Zoumenou

Key points

- Successful management of anaphylaxis relies upon rapid recognition and supportive treatment
- Awareness is common during general anesthesia (GA) for caesarean section and it is essential that there is adequate depth of anaesthesia throughout surgery
- Pregnant women are at risk of gastric aspiration during GA but can be minimized by greater use of regional anaesthesia
- All women for GA should have their airways assessed for potential difficult intubation
- The anaesthetic practitioner should have a well practiced algorithm for managing a difficult/failed intubation.

13.1 Anaphylaxis

True anaphylaxis is an IgE mediated reaction involving massive degranulation of mast cells or basophils releasing histamine, leucotrienes and other mediators of acute inflammation that requires prior exposure to the agent in question. However, the clinical presentation of a severe anaphylactoid reaction, which requires no prior exposure and is mediated through different pathways, is identical. The incidence of these severe reactions is approximately 1:10,000, is twice as frequent in women, and muscle relaxants are responsible for 60% of cases, although reactions to antibiotics, syntocinon, or chlorhexidine can occur. In 50% of cases, there has been no known prior exposure to the drug. Hypersensitivity to latex is becoming more common, and although the majority of cases result in dermatitis, in some studies latex is the second commonest cause of anaesthesia-related anaphylaxis.

The usual presentation is any combination of cardiovascular collapse, difficulty in ventilation because of bronchospasm leading to hypoxia, or a rash. If the patient is awake, there may be a cough. The reaction may be delayed by 15–30 minutes after exposure to the agent responsible, and not all of these signs need to be present for the clinical diagnosis to be made.

Anaphylaxis is a medical emergency and recovery depends on the early use of adrenaline and fluid resuscitation. However, some drugs, for example morphine, may cause smaller amounts of histamine release producing milder signs and symptoms.

13.1.1 Guidelines for the management of anaphylaxis

The Association of Anaesthetists of GB and Ireland have produced a sheet outlining the management of a patient with suspected anaphylaxis during anaesthesia, which may be downloaded from www.aagbi.org and attached to every anaesthetic machine.

13.1.1.1 *Primary treatment*

- Adopt an 'A, B, C' (Airway, Breathing, Circulation) approach
- Stop administration of the agent and call for help
- Give 100% oxygen and elevate patient's legs
- Intravenous fluids: crystalloid 2–4 litres, via large bore cannula
- Intravenous adrenaline.

An initial dose of adrenaline of 50mcg (0.5 ml of 1:10,000 solution) is appropriate for an adult. Subsequent doses of adrenaline will have to be titrated depending on the response. If 1 ml of a 1:10,000 solution is diluted to 10ml, the resulting 1:100,000 mixture contains 10mcg/ml adrenaline, which can be given in 1–5 ml increments, or by continuous infusion if necessary.

13.1.1.2 *Secondary treatment:*

If available, give IV chlorpheniramine 10mg and hydrocortisone 200mg. Additional treatment may be required for intractable bronchospasm.

If facilities exist for the estimation of plasma tryptase levels, blood samples (5–10 ml clotted blood) should be taken at the time of the reaction (do not delay resuscitation to take sample), after 1–2 hours, and at 24 hours. The samples should be spun to separate the serum/plasma and stored at 4° C if immediate analysis is possible or at −20° C for later analysis. A rise to >15mcg/l indicates probable anaphylaxis.

13.2 Awareness

Unintended intra-operative awareness occurs when a patient is conscious during some part of a general anaesthetic. The recall of events may be associated with pain and can lead to psychological problems. In the developed world, it occurs in about 1 in every 250 (4 per 1000) general anaesthetics for caesarean section, although vivid dreams may occur in as many as 6% of cases. An accurate figure for the developing world is not available. The risk can be minimized by careful attention to the details of the anaesthetic technique and observation of clinical signs of autonomic stimulation: tachycardia, hypertension, pupillary dilatation, lacrimation, and sweating. However, the cardiovascular signs can be caused by drugs such as atropine and ketamine and are not reliable predictors of awareness. The commonest causes of awareness are human error (administration of inadequate anaesthesia) or equipment failure (e.g. empty vaporiser).

The minimum alveolar concentration (MAC) of volatile anaesthetic agents is reduced in pregnancy by approximately 20%, and MAC awareness (the concentration at which 50% patients are awake rather than respond to a surgical stimulus) is thought to be about 0.5 of MAC. For these reasons the addition of, for example, 0.5% halothane to a 50:50 mixture of oxygen and nitrous oxide will help to significantly reduce the incidence of awareness.

The best way to establish the incidence of awareness is to ask four simple questions to all patients after recovery from general anaesthesia:

What was the last thing you remember before going to sleep?

What was the first thing you remember when you woke up?

Do you remember anything in between?

Did you have any unpleasant dreams?

A positive response to questions 3 or 4 will indicate the need for a more detailed interview.

Some patients experience post-traumatic stress disorder (PTSD), leading to long-lasting after-effects such as nightmares, night terrors, flashbacks, insomnia, and in some cases, even suicide. There is evidence that early psychological counselling and support can reduce the amount of harm and chances of developing PTSD.

If a patient has explicit recall of intra-operative events, it is important not to deny the existence of awareness, but treat them sympathetically and with compassion. Apologise to the patient and explain the fine balance between ensuring unconsciousness in the mother against the effects of excessive anaesthesia on the fetus and uterus.

13.3 Aspiration of gastric contents

The physiological changes of pregnancy place the mother at increased risk of aspiration of gastric contents during general anaesthesia. The consequences of pulmonary aspiration will depend on the volume and pH of the inhaled fluid, and whether it is particulate or not. In the most severe cases, the patient may develop a chemical pneumonitis with collapse and consolidation leading to hypoxia and an acute lung injury (Mendelson's syndrome). It is often associated with difficulty at intubation, but may equally well occur at tracheal extubation before the return of airway reflexes.

The patient may develop hypoxia, tachycardia, hypotension, bronchospasm, pulmonary oedema, and difficulty with ventilation. If the patient is extubated there will be tachypnoea and respiratory distress. The differential diagnosis of respiratory distress includes pulmonary embolism, amniotic fluid embolism, cardiac pulmonary oedema, asthma, and pneumothorax.

13.3.1 **Management**

Avoidance of general anaesthesia is the best way to prevent aspiration of gastric contents, although it may occur in women who have a depressed level of consciousness for other reasons such as after an eclamptic fit or hypoglycaemia. Other preventative measures involve reducing the volume and increasing the pH of gastric fluid. The most commonly used drugs are ranitidine (150mg orally every 6 hours in labour for those mothers deemed to be at high risk of requiring operative delivery) and sodium citrate (30 ml of 0.3 Molar solution given just before pre-oxygenation). Sodium citrate is preferred to particulate antacids such as magnesium trisilicate. For elective cases, patients should be starved for 6 hours before general anaesthesia and premedicated with ranitidine, but for urgent cases, gastric emptying will be delayed by pain or opioid analgesia and the stomach must always be assumed to be full. Consider using an orogastric tube to empty the stomach after delivery of the baby and before emergence.

13.3.2 **Treatment**

Regurgitation of gastric contents at induction:

- Tip patient head down
- Suction to pharynx (Yankauer)
- Intubate trachea
- Pass suction catheter down tracheal tube **before** ventilation (do not delay ventilation if patient is hypoxic)
- If significant volume is aspirated, postoperative ventilation may be necessary
- There is no evidence that prophylactic antibiotics and corticosteroids are effective. Antibiotics might be needed if secondary infection occurs
- Bronchodilators and diuretics for treatment of pulmonary oedema.

13.4 **Difficult and failed intubation**

Safe and successful airway management is a core, practical skill of all anaesthetists. It is also, unfortunately, the area of practice associated with the most avoidable mortality. Although the practical skill of tracheal intubation is central, safe airway management requires acquisition of skills in assessment, decision-making in the face of predictors of difficulty, use of airway adjuncts, face mask ventilation, and an understanding of steps to take in the event of failure. The incidence of failed intubation appears to be about 10 times higher in the obstetric population. An anaesthetist faced with a difficult or failed intubation should never hesitate to call for help.

13.4.1 **Airway assessment**

There are a number of different tests used to try to identify which patients will be difficult to intubate, but they all have relatively poor positive predictive values although reasonably high negative predictive values. What this means in practice is that not all patients who are predicted to be difficult will turn out to be difficult, but that almost everyone who is predicted to be easy will be easy. The airway assessment can, however, be used to formulate a plan for airway management.

The anatomical requirements for easy tracheal intubation are mouth opening, neck flexion, head extension at the cranio-cervical junction and a sub-mandibular space into which the tongue can move during laryngoscopy, and the airway assessment should test for these features. Conversely, any conditions that limit these features may result in difficulty, and the more predictors of difficulty that are present, the more likely it is that intubation will be difficult.

Table 13.1 Possible predictors of difficult intubation
• Previous history of difficult intubation
• Obesity
• Facial trauma, burns
• Temporomandibular joint (TMJ) limitation
• Arthritis restricting neck movement
• Protruding incisors
• Large/oedematous tongue
• Small mandible
• Submandibular infection/scarring/small space
• Short neck
• Previous tracheostomy

Table 13.2 Mallampati classification
1. Soft palate, uvula, fauces visible
2. Part of uvula, some posterior pharynx
3. Soft palate, base of uvula
4. Hard palate only

13.4.2 Simple tests

This is a rapid evaluation of the airway that takes less than one minute (the numbers refer to Table 13.3):

1. Ask the patient to open her mouth and stick out her tongue.

The Mallampati classification is an assessment of the view of soft tissue structures in the mouth, graded by what is visible with maximal opening and tongue protrusion but without phonation (Figure 13.1).

2. See how many fingers she can get between her upper and lower incisors. Assess prominence of incisors

3. Assess the range of movement of the head and neck from full flexion to full extension

4. Assess jaw slide by asking her to push her lower jaw forward

5. Assess the mandibular size and submandibular space by feeling between the thyroid cartilage and the chin.

The anaesthetist faced with a pregnant woman who is predicted to be difficult to intubate requiring an emergency caesarean section does not have very many options available. If more experienced help is available, they should be called, but even another pair of hands to help is useful. As an extreme example, consider a morbidly obese woman with a receding chin and limited mouth opening because of an anky-losed temporomandibular joint who has an antepartum haemorrhage causing hypotension and fetal distress. There are relative contra-indications to spinal anaesthesia, but general anaesthesia with muscle relaxation will almost certainly result in a failed intubation.

Where possible an algorithm for the management of difficult and failed intubation should be agreed locally, adapted for the equipment and experience that is available, and practised (Figure 13.2).

13.4.3 Explanation of algorithm

13.4.3.1 1st attempt

It is essential that everything is optimised so that the first attempt is the best attempt. Pay careful attention to the positioning of the head on a pillow, so that the neck is flexed and the head extended at the cranio-cervical junction. Ideally, the chin should be above the height

Table 13.3 Results of airway assessment		
Test	Normal	Possibly difficult
1	Class 1–2	Class 3–4
2	3 fingers/5 cm	< 3 fingers/5 cm
3	≥ 90°	< 90°
4	Lower incisors beyond upper incisors	Lower incisors do not reach upper incisors
5	Distance > 7 cm Soft tissues	Distance < 7 cm. Hard scarred tissues

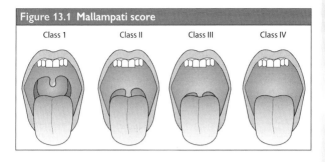

Figure 13.1 Mallampati score

Class 1   Class II   Class III   Class IV

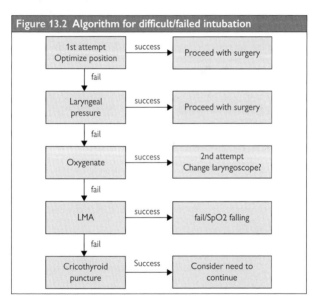

Figure 13.2 Algorithm for difficult/failed intubation

1st attempt
Optimize position —success→ Proceed with surgery

↓ fail

Laryngeal
pressure —success→ Proceed with surgery

↓ fail

Oxygenate —success→ 2nd attempt
Change laryngoscope?

↓ fail

LMA —success→ fail/SpO2 falling

↓ fail

Cricothyroid
puncture —Success→ Consider need to
continue

of the chest. Meticulous pre-oxygenation will provide the anaesthetist with as much time as possible before hypoxia occurs in the event of difficulty. If the larynx can be seen after induction of anaesthesia and muscle relaxation, proceed to intubate.

13.4.3.2 *Laryngeal pressure/bougie*

External laryngeal pressure may improve the view at laryngoscopy so that intubation can proceed. If only the epiglottis or arytenoid cartilages are visible it should be possible to place a bougie into the trachea and pass a tracheal tube over it. If the clicks of the tracheal rings are felt and the bougie meets resistance in the bronchi when *gently* advanced, it suggests it is in the trachea. If the bougie goes into the oesophagus, it tends to slide in easily without resistance. When advancing the tracheal tube over the bougie, rotate the tube 90° anticlockwise so that the bevel faces posteriorly as it passes through the glottis.

13.4.3.3 *Oxygenation*

If the first attempt fails, it may be necessary to re-oxygenate the mother before a second attempt. Alert the theatre staff that there is a problem and call for help if any is available. Insert a Guedel airway and consider four-hand ventilation (the anaesthetist uses two hands to hold the face mask and an assistant squeezes the reservoir or self-inflating bag). Minimize gastric insufflation.

13.4.3.4 *Second attempt*

Re-assess the patient's head position and optimize. Consider a different type of blade (e.g. McCoy or straight blade) if available and the anaesthetist is familiar with its use. If the second attempt fails, the priority is maternal oxygenation as above. Repeated attempts at intubation will cause trauma, swelling, bleeding and make subsequent mask ventilation more difficult. In addition, the mother will desaturate during the period of apnoea.

13.4.3.5 *Laryngeal mask airway*

If intubation and oxygenation by face mask both fail, insert a laryngeal mask airway (LMA). The correct size will depend on the woman's weight, but a size 4 will fit most women. Gently inflate the lungs with 100% oxygen so that there is no leak of air, because the LMA does not protect against regurgitation and aspiration of gastric contents.

13.4.3.6 *Consider the need to continue*

Once the mother is oxygenated, the decision has to be made about whether to continue with the caesarean section. This will be determined by a number of factors such as: elective case or emergency surgery for fetal distress, presence of bleeding, suitability for regional anaesthesia and type of muscle relaxant used. In principle, the mother's life takes priority over that of the fetus but in cases where a long acting relaxant has been used, or there is a significant antepartum haemorrhage, or a regional technique is contraindicated, then surgery has to continue under volatile or ketamine anaesthesia. Conversely, if it is an elective caesarean under general anaesthesia for maternal request and suxamethonium has been used, the mother should be woken up and a regional anaesthetic performed.

13.4.3.7 *Cricothyroid puncture*

If intubation and ventilation with face mask or LMA have both failed, the only way to oxygenate is via a cricothyroid puncture or tracheostomy. These techniques are associated with high morbidity, especially in untrained hands. A circuit consisting of a 14g cannula, three-way tap, oxygen tubing and a 15 mm tracheal tube connector can be used, but must be prepared beforehand (Figure 13.3). Puncture the cricothyroid membrane with the cannula, ensuring air can be aspirated from the trachea. Hold in place to avoid movement and kinking. Connect the three-way tap (with the side port open to air) and one end of the oxygen tubing, with the other end connected to the anaesthetic machine via the 15 mm connector. Use the emergency oxygen bypass to intermittently ventilate the lungs, making sure the upper airway is as patent as possible to allow air entrainment and exhalation. If there is no high-flow bypass, some ventilation may be achieved by intermittent occlusion of the side port of the three-way tap with maximal oxygen flow on the rotameter. It should be re-emphasized that this technique must only be used as a life-saving procedure.

Figure 13.3

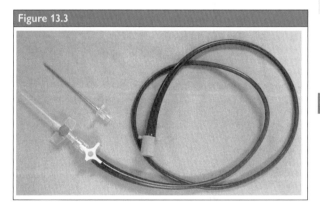

Chapter 14

Pre-existing disease

Raman Sivasankar, Sarah Harries

14.1 Human Immunodeficiency Virus (HIV)

> **Key points**
> - Anti-retroviral treatment from the second trimester to the postpartum period should be administered to all HIV infected mothers
> - Planned caesarean section is the safest mode of delivery if viral load is high
> - Six weeks zidovudine prophylaxis should be administered to all infants of mother sub-optimally treated during pregnancy
> - HIV is transmitted in breast milk.

The recent worldwide increase in antenatal HIV testing has resulted in more HIV infected women being diagnosed and cared for by clinicians during their pregnancy. Approximately 2.5 million children are living with HIV infection in the world. The vast majority acquired this disease via maternal to fetal vertical transmission.

14.1.1 Antenatal management

The care of a HIV positive mother starts in the antenatal period. All pregnant women must be tested for HIV infection early in pregnancy and positive results clearly recorded and communicated. A multidisciplinary team should oversee management, with an early assessment of social circumstances. During pregnancy, viral load, CD4 cell count and clinical status should be monitored regularly, as the results will dictate the safest mode of delivery for mother and baby. The mother should be regularly assessed for genitourinary and opportunistic infections and treated promptly.

14.1.2 Antiretroviral therapy (ART)

A combination of zidovudine (ZDV) and lamivudine should be commenced from second trimester through to the postpartum period.

The same drugs should be administered to babies for one week after delivery **OR** a single dose of nevirapine (NVP) administered in labour and then to the baby immediately after birth. ZDV monotherapy commenced by 28 weeks remains an acceptable option for women if the viral load is repeatedly <6-10000 HIV RNA copies/ml plasma, delivery is by planned caesarean section (CS), presence of wild type virus and the mother does not require highly active ART (HAART). In women presenting late for delivery, post exposure prophylaxis for the babies is advised, i.e. single dose of NVP and ZDV for the first six weeks of life. There is no evidence of any increase in congenital malformations to any ART to date; however, data for teratogenic risk is inadequate.

14.1.3 **Intrapartum management**

Measures to prevent mother to child transmission of HIV infection should be adopted. Planned CS is recommended for all women on ZDV monotherapy or combination therapy with detectable viraemia or HIV/Hepatitis C virus co-infection. CS should be planned for 38 weeks if on ZDV monotherapy **or** if viraemia is detected, or at 39 weeks if on HAART **and** viraemia not detected.

Vaginal delivery is an option if there is no viraemia and on HAART, but artificial rupture of membranes and invasive fetal monitoring should be avoided. Prolonged rupture of membranes is a risk factor for vertical transmission. Corticosteroids should be administered if preterm labour threatens or consider expedited delivery for pre-term rupture of membranes. Communication between team members is essential and delivery, by whatever mode, should be planned.

14.1.4 **Infant feeding**

Formula feeding avoids HIV transmission through breast milk and improves HIV free survival in infants. However, there is a higher infant mortality rate with formula feeds in rural African settings due to unhygienic practices. Exclusive breast feeding for 6 months would usually be advocated in poor socioeconomic settings, with prolonged infant ART to prevent transmission of infection through breast milk.

14.2.5 **Preconception advice**

The practice of self-insemination of partner's semen is safer than sexual intercourse and provides greater protection for the uninfected partner. Sperm washing prior to insemination has been recommended to offer further protection, but is very expensive.

14.2 Malaria

> ### Key points
> - Malaria infection in pregnancy leads to maternal anaemia and low infant birth weight
> - Regular antenatal visits should screen for anaemia and provide iron supplementation
> - WHO control strategies focus on intermittent preventative treatment, treated mosquito nets and effective case management in high transmission areas
> - Artemisinin combination therapy is effective against resistant falciparum malaria.

Malaria is an immense public health problem, with at least 50 million pregnant women living in malaria endemic areas. The two most important consequences of malaria in pregnancy are maternal anaemia and low infant birth weight.

In high transmission areas, plasmodium falciparum is prevalent in placental and peripheral blood. The prevalence is high in the first pregnancy and reduces as the parity increases, due to the acquisition of parity specific immunity. HIV and malaria co-infection reduces the immunity and delays clearance of parasites from the blood in multigravid women. In low transmission areas, the prevalence is less than 10% and hence there is reduced development of parity specific immunity. Plasmodium vivax infection is more common in primigravid women and is associated with poorer birth outcomes.

Control strategies for malaria in pregnancy depend upon the epidemiology of the infection. In high transmission areas, intermittent preventive treatment during pregnancy (IPTp), use of insecticide treated mosquito nets (ITNs) and case management are all advocated. In low transmission areas, case management is primarily emphasized.

14.2.1 Interventions for malaria control

The WHO recommended interventions for malaria control are as follows:
- Four antenatal visits with three after the first noted movements of the fetus
- ITN use from the first trimester through to the post partum period
- Two separate doses of IPTp with sulfadoxine-pyrimethamine (SP), first dose after start of fetal movements, second dose a month later. HIV positive women should receive three doses
- Effective case management of malaria
- Screening for anaemia and iron supplementation.

Weekly SP prophylaxis has been associated with rare but potentially fatal cutaneous reactions. However, the 2–4 doses of ITPp over 6 months has been well tolerated. Worsening of adverse drug reactions has been observed when ITPp of SP is used in HIV infected women receiving co-trimoxazole prophylaxis. High dose folic acid (5mg/day) interferes with antimalarial efficacy of SP and a dose of 0.4mg/day is recommended to prevent neural tube defects and maintain the effectiveness of SP.

14.2.2 Programme effectiveness

The issues that influence the effectiveness of the WHO programme are: gestational age of first visit, as the burden of malaria is higher if the treatment starts late; attendance of adolescents who have a poorer outcome; and increased distance from the main district hospitals, as this usually indicates less opportunities for education and referral.

14.2.3 Treatment

Malarial parasites are resistant to the traditional anti-malarial drug chloroquine, therefore, the WHO recommends for treatment artemisinin combination therapy (ACT) for uncomplicated falciparum malaria. The choice of ACT depends on the resistance in the geographical region and must be given for at least 3 days:

- In Southeast Asia—artesunate-mefloquine or artemether-lumefantrine
- In Africa—artemether-lumefantrine or artesunate-amodiaquine or artesunate-sulfadoxine & pyrimethamine (SP).

In the first trimester, quinine and clindamycin should be given for 7 days or quinine monotherapy, if clindamycin is unavailable; however, ACT should be used in the second and third trimester. ACT can be used in the first trimester if it is the only effective treatment available.

Lactating mothers can safely receive all antimalarials except for tetracycline and dapsone.

14.3 Anaemia

Key points

- Anaemia (Hb <11 gm/dl) in pregnancy is associated with increased risks to both mother and infant
- Underlying helminthiasis infection should be excluded or treated
- Iron plus folate replacement therapy is more effective than iron therapy alone.

Severe anaemia in pregnancy is associated with increased risk of maternal and perinatal mortality, low infant birth weight, infant iron deficiency anaemia and adverse behavioral and cognitive development in children.

Anaemia is defined as a haemoglobin (Hb) concentration of less than 11 gm/dl and severe anaemia is less than 7 gm/dl. The main causes of anaemia include: iron deficiency, malaria, helminthiasis, HIV infection, sickle cell disease, and haemoglobinopathies. The following factors also contribute to anaemia in pregnancy: adolescent or concealed pregnancy, late antenatal booking, grand multi-parity and other nutritional deficiencies e.g. folate, vitamins A and B 12. A vegetarian diet is low in iron and the phytates in cereals interfere with iron absorption.

The body of healthy adult women contains 3.5–4.5 grams of iron, of which 75% is in red blood cells as haemoglobin, 20% as ferritin in the bone marrow and reticulo-endothelial system and 5% in muscle and the enzyme system. Anaemia is usually asymptomatic; however, it may present with fatigue and/or dyspnoea.

14.3.1 Treatment

The mainstay of treatment is oral replacement with ferrous sulphate 200mg three times per day, plus folic acid 5mg once daily.

Iron plus folate is more effective than iron alone, irrespective of serum folate levels. Hb is expected to rise at least 0.2 gm/dl per week. If not, other causes of anaemia have to be explored and treated.

In hookworm endemic regions, antenatal antihelminthics have been shown to reduce the incidence of low birth weight and improve infant survival. Helminthic infection is treated with mebendazole 500mg orally or albendazole 400mg orally, both as a single dose after the first trimester.

14.4 Cardiac disease

Key points

- Rheumatic mitral stenosis is the most common cause of death related to cardiac disease in Africa
- Regular antenatal monitoring will assist in the diagnosis of the mother with progressive cardiac disease prompting optimization of her cardiac condition or early delivery
- During labour, stress on the mother and her heart should be minimized, whilst cardiac output and fetal perfusion is maintained

> ### Key points (*Contd.*)
> - Effective pain relief in labour will minimize cardiac work
> - Regional techniques are safe in the parturient with cardiac disease, except for those with a fixed cardiac output
> - It is the care with which the anaesthetic technique is performed that is more important than the choice of technique
> - Oxytocin causes profound hypotension and tachycardia - it should be administered as a slow IV bolus over 5-10 minutes
> - Overzealous fluid replacement can precipitate pulmonary oedema, which can be fatal
> - Critical care monitoring should be continued for 48hours after delivery, as cardiac complications can present at a later stage.

Heart disease in pregnancy is highly prevalent in developing countries and causes an unacceptably high morbidity and mortality. The National Committee on Confidential Enquiries into Maternal Deaths (NCCEDM) reported that close to half of non-obstetric maternal deaths in South Africa were due to cardiac disease. The report identified the causes and several preventable factors that precipitated decompensation and maternal mortality.

14.4.1 Causes
The following causes of underlying cardiac disease are prevalent in the developing world: rheumatic heart disease, valvular heart disease, infective endocarditis, AIDS related puerperal cardiomyopathy, congenital heart disease, peripartum cardiomyopathy, and ischaemic heart disease. The most common cause of death is secondary to rheumatic mitral stenosis, where the mortality can be reduced by adequate medical care.

14.4.2 Preventable factors
There are a number of preventable factors which contribute to a poor outcome for mother and baby. The increase in cardiac output during labour presents an enormous challenge for a mother with pre-existing cardiac disease. Labour pain must be managed effectively to limit the surge in catecholamines during contractions, which will inevitably lead to cardiac compromise. Inadvertent intravenous fluid overload and a lack of awareness of the increase in blood volume that occurs at placental separation both contribute to cardiac failure in the first 24 hours following delivery. Inadequate assessment of a woman during the early stages of cardiac decompensation often leads to increased complications. In resource poor countries, patient's often seek medical attention very late or only *in extremis* making the management of cardiac disease extremely difficult or

beyond treatment. This is a problem for those women living remotely, who receive inadequate or no antenatal care.

14.4.3 **Valvular heart disease**

Although any valvular heart lesion can present for the first time during pregnancy, mitral stenosis related to previous rheumatic fever is the most commonly observed in the developing world. Most other valve disease is congenitally acquired in isolation or as part of a more complex congenital cardiac problem.

Rheumatic mitral stenosis is caused by mitral valve leaflet thickening and calcification, commissural fusion, chordal fusion or a combination of these processes. The mitral valve is normally 4–5 cm^2. Symptoms develop when the valve area is reduced to 2.5 cm^2 and an area more than 1.5 cm^2 does not produce symptoms at rest. As the valve area decreases the transmitral pressure gradient increases and the increasing pressure is reflected back into the pulmonary circulation. In chronic mitral stenosis, the pulmonary arterioles develop intimal hyperplasia and medial hypertrophy, which leads to pulmonary arterial hypertension. Mitral stenosis (MS) is a continuous, progressive disease with a slow stable course in the early years, followed by a progressive acceleration in later life. The first symptoms of dyspnoea in mild MS are associated with exercise, emotional stress, pregnancy, infection and atrial fibrillation with a rapid ventricular response.

14.4.3.1 *Diagnosis*

Physical examination will confirm an early diastolic heart murmur, often with a small volume, irregular pulse. ECG features are of secondary atrial fibrillation (AF). The diagnosis is confirmed on echocardiogram.

14.4.3.2 *Management*

Management includes rheumatic fever prophylaxis with penicillins, negative chronotropic agents, e.g. digoxin, beta blockers to treat AF, salt restriction and diuretics, infective endocarditis prophylaxis, anticoagulation if AF present, followed by planned mitral valvotomy or mitral valve replacement as resources allow.

14.4.3.3 *Patient counselling*

It is essential that the mother is monitored antenatally for any signs of worsening valve disease and is encouraged to seek medical attention if/when symptoms deteriorate. Contraception is strongly recommended in severe MS until valvular surgery is complete.

14.4.4 **AIDS related cardiomyopathy**

Myocardial disease is the most important cardiovascular manifestation of HIV infection. It may present as myocarditis, dilated cardiomyopathy or isolated left or right ventricular dysfunction. The causes for the myocardial involvement are multifactorial: myocardial invasion with HIV, opportunistic infection, viral infection, autoimmune response to viral infection, drug related cardiac toxicity, nutritional deficiency, and prolonged immunosuppression. The myocardial involvement can cause symptomatic cardiac failure. Highly active antiretroviral therapy (HAART) has significantly reduced the incidence of cardiovascular involvement.

14.4.5 **Cardiomyopathy**

There are two types of cardiomyopathy, dilated, which includes peripartum cardiomyopathy and hypertrophic obstructive cardiomyopathy.

14.4.5.1 *Peripartum cardiomyopathy (PPCM)*

PPCM can present as congestive cardiac failure in the last month of pregnancy or the first five months postpartum. It often presents when there is no history of pre-existing cardiac disease. It is diagnosed on an echocardiogram with severely impaired left ventricular function. Maternal mortality is very high, only half of women with PPCM make a complete recovery. Treatment options include diuretics, intravenous nitrate infusion and inotropes, e.g. dobutamine or enoximone.

14.4.5.2 *Hypertrophic obstructive cardiomyopathy (HOCM)*

This is a genetically transmitted cardiac disease, often presenting as sudden death in adolescence. It has a prevalence of 1 in 500–1,000. The underlying condition leads to asymmetrical myocardial hypertrophy.

14.4.6 **Ischaemic heart disease**

In the developed world, the prevalence of ischaemic heart disease in women of child-bearing years has increased in recent years due to lifestyle changes, e.g. increased smoking, obesity, stress, and older women conceiving. The developing world may see a similar pattern emerging in future generations. Acute coronary syndrome in pregnancy is very rare, but the morbidity and mortality are very high.

14.4.7 **Management of mothers with cardiac disease**

The management of the mothers with cardiac disease starts in the preconception phase and continues throughout the pregnancy and postpartum period. Preconception planning will optimize the cardiovascular system in preparation for the pregnancy.

14.4.7.1 *Preconception*

Any woman with an underlying cardiac disease should be optimized prior to conception to minimize the risk of cardiovascular disease progression during pregnancy, e.g. planned valvotomy for rheumatic mitral stenosis, or counselled about the potential risks of pregnancy and delivery for her and her baby. Any current drug treatment should be reviewed and changed to the safest drug regime for early pregnancy e.g. use of heparin instead of warfarin, avoidance of ACE inhibitors. Nutritional advice should be given and anaemia treated.

14.4.7.2 *Antenatal care*

Cardiac output increases by 40% and blood volume increases by 50% by 20 weeks of pregnancy. Systemic vascular resistance (SVR) falls, which may lead to reversal of an existing left-right cardiac shunt e.g. persistent ventricular septal defect. These cardiovascular changes cause rapid decompensation, but are usually heralded by fatigue, shortness of breath and inability to cope with normal daily activities. Assessment during the antenatal period should be based on the functional New York Heart Association classification and reassessed as pregnancy progresses.

- NYHA 1—No limit during ordinary activity
- NYHA 2—Slight limitation during ordinary activity
- NYHA 3—Marked limitation of ordinary activity
- NYHA 4—No physical activity without symptoms.

If symptoms are detected at this early stage, women can be offered the support required i.e. hospital admission for optimization of medical treatment, possible surgical intervention to prolong pregnancy or early delivery of baby. A multidisciplinary approach to patient care is vital, including the obstetrician, anaesthetist, cardiologist, and midwife.

14.4.7.3 *Intra-partum care*

Labour and vaginal delivery

The primary aim during labour is to reduce the stress on the mother and her heart, whilst maintaining cardiac output, placental, and fetal circulation. Effective pain relief is therefore essential. Where resources are available, the ideal technique would be a low dose epidural for the duration of labour e.g. 0.1% bupivacaine and 2mcg/ml fentanyl as 5 ml slow incremental boluses to provide analgesia with minimal haemodynamic disturbance.

Caesarean section

A variety of anaesthetic techniques have been described for the management of a mother with cardiac disease; epidural anaesthesia, a low dose combined spinal-epidural technique, spinal catheter with incremental top-ups or general anaesthesia. The technique performed will depend on the available resources; however, any technique should be used cautiously in the high-risk cardiac mother with the provision for invasive arterial BP monitoring and/or central venous pressure (CVP) monitoring. Regional techniques are considered safe for most cardiac conditions, except for fixed cardiac output states, providing haemodynamic stability is maintained with appropriate use of vasopressors and relief of aorto-caval compression.

The care with which each technique is performed is more important than the technique itself, as the choice of technique can be influenced by many factors. As a general principle, regional anaesthetic techniques are relatively contra-indicated in a parturient with a fixed cardiac output i.e. moderate to severe aortic stenosis, although in experienced hands it is now considered a safe option.

Haemorrhage

Any degree of blood loss in the mother with cardiac disease should be managed with great thought and care. She will have reduced capacity to compensate for hypovolaemia if she has a fixed cardiac output, e.g. aortic stenosis or HOCM, any expected compensatory tachycardia can be obtunded by beta-blocker drugs or cardiac conduction abnormalities and overzealous intravenous fluid infusion can rapidly result in pulmonary oedema. Institute regular monitoring of pulse, BP, oxygen saturations and urine output regardless of measured blood loss. Replace intravenous fluids in 250–500ml increments and reassess the mother regularly. Pulmonary oedema should be treated promptly with oxygen and diuretics.

Pulmonary oedema

Pulmonary oedema in parturients with cardiac disease can be due to excessive intravenous fluid replacement, autotransfusion of blood from the contracting uterus, sever pre-eclampsia or left ventricular failure. Furosemide 20–40mg at the time of delivery may help counteract the effects of autotransfusion from the uterus.

Oxytocics

Oxytocin causes a significant decrease in the systemic vascular resistance and mean arterial pressure, and an increase in heart rate after administration. These haemodynamic changes are easily tolerated by healthy parturients but not by those with cardiac disease. Avoiding oxytocin is not an option, as it will lead to major haemorrhage but it should be administered with great care, e.g. dilute 5 IU in 20 ml saline and administer over 5–10 minutes, followed by 40 IU in 500 ml saline over 4–6 hours.

Ergometrine is a powerful uterotonic, but associated with hypertension, pulmonary vasoconstriction and profound nausea and vomiting. Ergometrine (500mcg) can be given in combination with oxytocin (5 units) as an intramuscular injection in mild to moderate cardiac disease, but not in severe cardiac disease or in the presence of pulmonary or systemic hypertension.

Uterine massage, an intrauterine balloon and a B-lynch suture performed prophylactically at an elective caesarean section can assist in the control of postpartum haemorrhage.

Arrythmias

Arrythmias can impair cardiac filling, cardiac output and coronary perfusion. Drugs that cause a tachycardia, e.g. ephedrine, atropine, oxytocin should be avoided or given as a titrated IV bolus to women who have a history of tachyarrythmias. Phenylephrine is the vasoconstrictor of choice in regional anaesthesia.

Embolism

Many patients with cardiac disease are at high risk of thromboembolism and may be treated with prophylactic or therapeutic doses of anticoagulants. Any clotting abnormalities or recent dosing of anticoagulants should be carefully considered before performing a regional anaesthetic procedure (see Chapter 7).

Women with intra-cardiac shunts are at increased risk of paradoxical air embolism and extreme care must be taken to avoid air bubbles in the intravenous line.

Bacterial endocarditis

Any parturient with a history of valvular heart disease, cardiac surgery or infective endocarditis should be administered prophylactic antibiotics to reduce the risk of recurrent endocarditis:

- amoxicillin 1 gm and gentamicin 120mg given intravenously at delivery, followed by amoxicillin 500mg six hours later is an essential part of peripartum care.

Postpartum care

Critical care monitoring of vital signs should continue for at least 48–72 hours into the post partum period, as risk of cardiac complications persist. Meticulous attention to fluid balance is essential and post-delivery analgesia and thrombo-prophylaxis should be prescribed and administered. Be watchful for the development of co-incidental pre-eclampsia, pulmonary oedema, respiratory complications such as aspiration pneumonitis, basal atelectasis, or pneumonia. Anti-retroviral therapy should be administered to both mother and baby if required, and the infant should be screened for congenital cardiac disease.

Chapter 15

The sick mother

Saira Hussain, Sarah Harries

Key points

- It is important to recognize the sick mother by vigilant monitoring of basic parameters
- Early detection of clinical deterioration is helped by the use of an early warning score
- Good critical care depends on basic monitoring and appropriately trained staff employing locally generated protocols and is possible in a low resource setting
- Peripartum caesarean section may save the maternal life
- Successful management of maternal trauma depends upon prompt assessment and treatment.

15.1 Recognition

Serious illness arising during pregnancy or the puerperium may be difficult to recognize because of altered maternal physiology. The rapid administration of oxygen and intravenous fluids may be lifesaving and initial efforts should be directed to maintaining oxygenation and perfusion of vital organs whilst the underlying cause is looked for. Various factors in the woman's medical or obstetric history may provide clues to the diagnosis and a look, listen, feel approach can demonstrate signs in the absence of sophisticated monitoring equipment.

15.1.1 Signs of serious illness

Regular charting of vital signs may help identify those women who are deteriorating and an early warning scoring system will highlight this (see Table 15.1). The score from each parameter is added together to give a total score. A woman whose overall score is rising needs urgent medical assessment.

Figure 15.1 is an example early warning chart where abnormal parameters are readily identified when recordings lie in the coloured zones. The nurse should inform the doctor when the patient triggers pale blue, or two gray scores at any one time. A moderate alert gives a score of one and a high alert give a score of two.

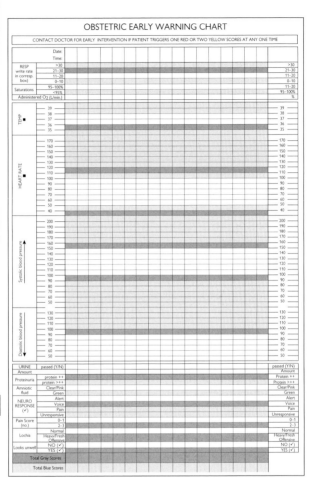

Figure 15.1 Early Warning Observation Chart. Parameters are recorded on a regular basis by nursing or midwifery staff. The ideal colours are yellow for moderate alert and red for high alert. In this example yellow is replaced by gray, and red by pale blue. Adapted version of original MEWS chart, reprinted with permission from Dr. Fiona McIlveney, Dr. Chris Cairns and colleagues from Stirling Royal Infirmary.

15.1.1.1 *Indicative physical signs*

Increased respiratory rate or tachypnoea is always a worrying sign and should never be ignored. It may indicate hypovolaemia, sepsis, or a respiratory cause. Tachycardia may indicate hypovolaemia, cardiac

Table 15.1 Early Warning Scoring System for the obstetric Patient

Score	2	1	0	1	2
Resps	<10		11–20	21–30	>30
Temp		<36	36–38		>38
HR	<40	40-50	51–100	101–120	>120
Systolic BP	<90	90-100	100–150	151–160	>160
Diastolic BP			40–90	90–100	>100
Proteinuria				++	>++
Amniotic Fluid			Clear/pink		Green
CNS	P or U	V	A		
Pain Score			0–1	2–3	
Lochia			Normal	Heavy/offensive	

Resps=respirations per minute, Temp=temperature, HR=heart rate, CNS=central nervous system, A=alert, V=responds to voice, P=responds to pain, U=unconscious, Pain score 0=no pain, 1=mild pain, 2=moderate pain, 3=severe pain

Score 0 equals low risk

Score 1 equals moderate risk

Score 2 equals high risk and action required.

failure, or an arrhythmia. The pulse may be weak or thready in each case. If the pulse is full volume and bounding, with warm hands and feet, consider sepsis as the cause. Poor urine output can indicate poor renal perfusion due to hypovolaemia. Urine output should equate to at least 0.5 ml/kg/hr or at least 100 ml in 4 hours. See Table 15.1.

15.2 Resuscitation

Initial resuscitation efforts aim to prevent vital organ damage by restoring adequate tissue perfusion using supplemental oxygen, as well as supporting the circulation with intravenous fluids. Control of haemorrhage and early administration of antibiotics may also be considered as part of the resuscitation process.

Follow an ABC (Airway, Breathing, Circulation) approach. Never progress from A to B, etc. until each problem is resolved, and reassess regularly for any signs of improvement after intervention until the patient is stable. Call for help early on and use electronic monitoring if available. See Table 15.2.

Table 15.2 ABC action plan		
	Problem	**Action**
Airway (put vertical to reduce space)	Absence of breath sounds or noisy breathing	Head tilt, chin lift, jaw thrust. Suction (only suck what you can see—never insert an instrument far back into the throat blindly otherwise the patient may gag and vomit). Use oropharyngeal or nasopharyngeal airway if available. Assist respirations if necessary with a self inflating bag, pocket mask or rescuer breaths and consider intubation if above manoeuvres are unsuccessful. Apply high flow oxygen once airway established. Turn into the recovery position if airway patent but conscious level depressed.
Breathing	Respiratory rate < 10 or > 25 breaths/min or cyanosis. In dark skinned people cyanosis is most apparent in the mucous membranes and nail beds.	Administer high flow oxygen, seek immediate treatable cause, e.g. pneumothorax, drug overdose, exacerbation of asthma. Consider intubation if becoming exhausted or unable to improve respiratory pattern.
Circulation	Heart rate > 100beat/min or > systolic blood pressure, systolic BP < 100, weak or absent peripheral pulses (absent radial = systolic of 90 or less, absent brachial = 80 or less and absent carotid = 60 or less), capillary refill time > 2 secs, < 100 ml urine in 4 hours.	Manually displace the gravid uterus to the left, establish IV access and give fluid boluses of 500 ml as necessary. Control haemorrhage by bimanual compression, oxytocic drugs or surgical intervention. Consider antibiotic therapy in sepsis. If available, monitor heart rhythm or perform ECG.
Disability	Altered mental status, unequal, pinpoint or dilated pupils or seizures.	High flow oxygen and recovery position. Palpate pulse and check BP—if weak and thready administer a fluid bolus. Consider immediate treatable cause, e.g. naloxone for opioid overdose. Check blood sugar levels and administer 25–50 ml 50% dextrose if <2. If hypertensive, hyperreflexic or 3+ beats of clonus, consider magnesium sulphate 4 g bolus over 5 minutes followed by infusion. If responsive to pain only or unresponsive, definitive airway protection is necessary.

15.3 **Basic critical care**

Critical care during pregnancy may require only monitoring, fluids and oxygen. However, some women may require more intensive support such as ventilation or renal replacement therapy. Best use should be made of locally available drugs, equipment, and trained personnel and the availability of these local resources will dictate the level of care provision for the critically ill woman. Vital signs should be recorded regularly on a standardized chart.

> **Suggested minimum observations to chart hourly or more frequently if the patient is unstable**
> Pulse rate
> Respiratory rate
> Blood pressure (or presence/absence carotid/femoral/radial pulses)
> Oxygen saturations (cyanosis/pallor)
> Capillary refill time
> Fluid input/intake
> Urine output
> Conscious level (AVPU = Alert, responds to Voice, responds to Pain, Unconscious).
> Pupils
> Antepartum PV loss
> Lochia (amount/colour/smell)

Regardless of the available local resources, there are basic principles of critical care that should always be adhered to.

15.3.1 **Infection**

Critically ill patients are immunocompromised, therefore it is essential to minimize the risk of infection. An apron and clean gloves should be worn before touching each patient whenever there is a risk of contact with body fluids, e.g. sputum or blood. Clean water and soap solution should be available to ensure hand washing by staff between patients. Patients with active respiratory or gastrointestinal infections should be isolated or nursed separately from other patients. Ideally, equipment should be single use or there should be adequate facilities for ensuring that it can be cleaned or sterilized appropriately. There should be an adequate amount of space between beds, and visitors should be encouraged to observe infection control procedures.

15.3.2 **Position**

Pregnant patients should be nursed with a degree of left uterine displacement to minimize the effect of aortocaval compression, e.g.

with a pillow or wedge. If this is not possible, the woman should be nursed in the full left lateral position. The intubated patient should have a degree of head up tilt (30°) to prevent pooling of secretions around the tracheal tube cuff. Suctioning through the tracheal tube should be performed regularly to prevent stagnation and infection of secretions.

15.3.3 Nutrition

Severe illness is a catabolic state with the breakdown of muscle providing energy and nutrients, and pregnancy itself increases calorie requirements to approximately 40 kcal/kg/day. Muscle weakness and nutritional deficiencies can greatly hinder or prolong recovery and contribute to morbidity. Adequate nutrition is also essential to reduce infection and provide the necessary nutrients for adequate wound healing. Ideally, nutrition should be by the enteral route. Patients should be encouraged to eat and drink, but if this is not possible, feeding should be established or supplemented via a nasogastric tube with nutritionally balanced products. Enteral feeding maintains the integrity of the gut mucosa and can reduce bacterial gut translocation as a source of systemic sepsis.

15.3.4 Thrombo-embolic prophylaxis

Pregnancy is a hypercoagulable state and critical illness is an independent risk factor for the development of venous thrombo-embolism. Other contributory factors include immobility, ileo-femoral vein compression, major surgery and pre-existing illness. Ideally, thromboprophylaxis, e.g. heparin 5000 iu or enoxaparin 20–40mg by subcutaneous injection, should be given appropriate to the stage of pregnancy. In the absence of anticoagulant drugs, compression stockings, and early mobilization can also reduce the risk.

15.4 Cardiac arrest and peri-mortem CS

Cardiac arrest may occur due to an acute exacerbation of a pre-existing illness or as a consequence of pregnancy or delivery, for example haemorrhage.

15.4.1 Cardiac arrest (see Figure 15.2)

In a woman who has collapsed and is unresponsive:

- *Open the airway* with a head tilt, chin lift manoeuvre. Jaw thrust may be necessary. Use an oro/nasopharyngeal airway and suction to clear secretions/blood/vomit/foreign body
- *Displace the gravid uterus* manually, or tilt the woman into the left lateral position to reduce aortocaval compression. Use a pillow or a wedge or ask someone to manually displace the uterus upwards and to the left. Elevate the legs to improve venous return

- If there are no signs of life after opening the airway, commence cardiopulmonary resuscitation—30 chest compressions to 2 ventilations and follow ALS algorithm (Figure 15.2)
- *Cannulate and administer an IV fluid bolus.* Attach defibrillation paddles if available, assess cardiac rhythm and treat according to ALS
- *Ventilate* with the highest concentration of oxygen available—this may require mouth to mouth, mouth to nose, pocket mask or bag-valve mask ventilation. The airway should be secured with a cuffed tracheal tube and cricoid pressure maintained until this is achieved
- *Intubation* may be more difficult in the pregnant patient due to airway oedema and so a smaller cuffed tracheal tube should be used. A gum elastic bougie may be useful. It should be remembered that due to the higher basal metabolic rate and reduced functional residual capacity that desaturation will occur rapidly
- *Chest compressions* should be performed slightly higher on the sternum in the pregnant woman and once the airway is secured should be performed continuously at a rate of 100 per minute. Approximately 12 ventilatory breaths per minute should be given
- *Check for and correct* any reversible cause of cardiac arrest
- 4 Hs = hypoxia, hypovolaemia, hypo/hyperkalaemia, hypothermia
- 4 Ts = tension pneumothorax, tamponade, thromboembolism, toxic/therapeutic disturbances.

If the cardiac output is still absent after 4 minutes of resuscitation, consider emergency caesarean section. This will relieve aorto-caval compression and may be life saving.

15.4.2 **Perimortem caesarean section**

This should be performed before the fifth minute of cardiac arrest by the most experienced obstetrician available for speed.

The primary aim of perimortem caesarean section is to facilitate maternal resuscitation by removing a potential cause of aortocaval compression and also the physiological burden of a non-vital organ i.e. the fetus. The secondary aim is to attempt salvage of a viable fetus when maternal resuscitation is futile.

15.4.2.1 *Procedure*

- Cardiopulmonary resuscitation should be ongoing—trans-abdominal cardiac massage may also be performed at laparotomy
- A long midline incision from the xiphoid process to the pubis should be performed passing through the skin and abdominal layers
- A vertical incision is made through the upper segment of the uterus
- The fetus is removed for resuscitation, the umbilical cord clamped and the placenta removed.

If maternal resuscitation is likely to be futile, rapid closure of the layers is acceptable. If there is maternal improvement, careful closure of all layers is essential as bleeding points may only be obvious once adequate cardiac output is restored. A coagulopathy may develop. Antibiotic prophylaxis is essential as the surgery is likely to be 'dirty'.

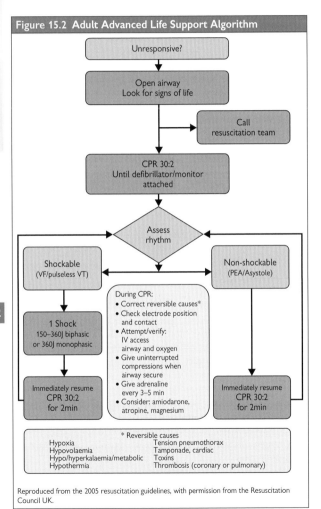

Figure 15.2 Adult Advanced Life Support Algorithm

Unresponsive?

Open airway
Look for signs of life

Call resuscitation team

CPR 30:2
Until defibrillator/monitor attached

Assess rhythm

Shockable
(VF/pulseless VT)

Non-shockable
(PEA/Asystole)

1 Shock
150–360J biphasic
or 360J monophasic

During CPR:
- Correct reversible causes*
- Check electrode position and contact
- Attempt/verify:
  IV access
  airway and oxygen
- Give uninterrupted compressions when airway secure
- Give adrenaline every 3–5 min
- Consider: amiodarone, atropine, magnesium

Immediately resume
CPR 30:2
for 2min

Immediately resume
CPR 30:2
for 2min

* Reversible causes

Hypoxia	Tension pneumothorax
Hypovolaemia	Tamponade, cardiac
Hypo/hyperkalaemia/metabolic	Toxins
Hypothermia	Thrombosis (coronary or pulmonary)

Reproduced from the 2005 resuscitation guidelines, with permission from the Resuscitation Council UK.

15.5 **Sepsis**

Intrapartum and postpartum infection is a significant cause of morbidity and mortality for mother, fetus, and neonate. It is responsible for around 25% of deaths in low income countries. Sub-clinical, ascending infections through the lower female genital tract are predominant worldwide but are more prevalent in low income countries.

15.5.1 **Definitions**

Sepsis is considered present if infection is highly suspected or proven and two or more of the following systemic inflammatory response syndrome (SIRS) criteria are met:

- Heart rate > 90 bpm
- Body temperature < 36 °C (96.8 °F) or > 38 °C (100.4 °F)
- Respiratory rate > 20 breaths per minute or a $PaCO_2$ less than 32 mm Hg (4.3 kPa)
- White blood cell count < 4000 cells/mm³ or > 12000 cells/mm³ (< 4 x 109 or > 12 x 109 cells/L), or greater than 10% band forms (immature white blood cells).

Septic shock is defined as hypotension, in the presence of sepsis, unresponsive to fluid resuscitation with evidence of compromised organ perfusion. Symptoms such as vomiting, diarrhoea, abdominal pain may occur in the absence of fever. Prompt recognition and treatment is essential as clinical deterioration may be rapid and overwhelming.

15.5.2 **Obstetric sepsis**

Obstetric sepsis most commonly occurs peri-partum or after abortion, and is due to a combination of aerobic and anaerobic organisms. It usually occurs as a result of ascending pathogens from the vagina or cervix. Infection may be more severe in the immuno-compromised, e.g. HIV mother.

15.5.3 **Underlying causes**

- *Obstetric-related:* Chorioamnionitis/endometritis, after incomplete or illegal abortion or following retained products of conception. Postpartum endometritis is common after vaginal delivery in low income countries. Wound infection and necrotizing fasciitis may occur after episiotomy or caesarean section
- *Non-obstetric:* Pneumonia, pyelonephritis, cholecystitis and other intra-abdominal foci.

15.5.4 **Treatment**

Treatment involves optimizing oxygen delivery and supporting organ perfusion using oxygen, intravenous fluids and vasopressors such as noradrenaline or adrenaline, and broad spectrum antibiotic therapy.

A typical antibiotic regimen for pelvic sepsis includes penicillin or ampicillin, gentamicin, and clindamycin or metronidazole. Sepsis due to tetanus remains a cause of mortality after septic abortion.

Heart rate, blood pressure, urine output, temperature, oxygen saturations, conscious level should all be monitored as well as strict attention to fluid input/output. If available, central venous pressure monitoring may be used to guide fluid management.

Drainage or debridement of infected or necrotic tissue/curettage to remove retained products/radiologically guided drainage of abscesses or laparotomy pockets of infection is absolutely essential for removal of the septic focus.

Delivery may be necessary if there is unresolved chorioamnionitis but sepsis may cause disseminated intravascular coagulation and this should be considered prior to operative intervention.

15.5.5 Other considerations

Reduced organ perfusion in maternal sepsis will result in uteroplacental insufficiency and fetal compromise or the onset of preterm labour. Expedited delivery of the fetus may be required if the mother remains seriously ill, as evacuation of the uterus may improve maternal haemodynamics.

15.6 Trauma

Trauma is an important cause of morbidity and mortality in the developing world. Poverty and poor infrastructure can increase risk of injury through road traffic accidents or unsafe living environments. Domestic violence or violent crime is common in socially eroded or unstable societies.

The best chance for a successful outcome of an injured mother and her fetus relies on prompt assessment and treatment of maternal life-threatening injuries by skilled practitioners.

15.6.1 Mechanisms of injury

15.6.1.1 *Blunt trauma*

- *Road Traffic Accidents* All types of injury may occur either as a pedestrian or a passenger/driver in a vehicle. Seat belts should be worn but should be positioned correctly to avoid blunt abdominal injury. The lap belt should pass beneath her abdomen resting on the anterior superior iliac spine and pubis with a shoulder strap between the breasts. Deceleration forces during a collision may cause neck injury as well as insidious internal damage to thoraco-abdominal structures with little or no evidence of external damage. Uterine rupture and direct fetal damage may result from major collisions. Shear forces may cause placental separation and abruption which may occur up to 48 hours after the accident

- *Falls* Hormonal changes in pregnancy causes ligamentous relaxation of the pelvic joints and spine, and the enlarging gravid uterus alters the centre of gravity. Pregnancy and lactation in combination with poor diet results in bone demineralization allowing fractures to occur more easily
- *Physical Abuse* Usually directed at the abdomen and genitalia. Often repetitive and sustained as victims do not often seek help.

15.6.1.2 *Penetrating injury*

Gunshot and Stab Wounds Injury to the upper abdomen is more likely to result in damage to the small bowel, liver or spleen as the gravid uterus displaces the abdominal organs upward. Injury to the lower abdomen may cause uterine and fetal damage. Traumatic penetration of the uterus is associated with 67% fetal death rate. Debris may be carried deep into the wound by bullets, pellets or shrapnel or via dirty implements increasing risk of infection and tissue necrosis.

15.6.2 **Obstetric injury**

The signs and symptoms of hypovolaemia may not occur until 30–40% of circulating blood volume has been lost. Ongoing bleeding will result in haemostatic failure as clotting factors are consumed. Damage to uterine vessels can cause rapid haemorrhage due to increased flow rates of up to 600 ml per minute. There may be concealed retroperitoneal bleeding from pelvic fracture or pelvic vessel disruption. Pelvic fracture also makes the fetus more susceptible to direct injury.

Aortocaval compression will worsen an already compromised cardiac output and must be relieved by lateral displacement of the uterus. Maternal catecholamine release during trauma will cause sympathetically mediated vasoconstriction of the uteroplacental circulation and will compromise fetal oxygenation. Uterine irritability, membrane rupture, and labour may occur as a result of direct injury or release of hormonal mediators in response to trauma. There may be loss of liquor, cord prolapse or ascending infection causing chorioamnionitis. Tocolysis (uterine relaxation) should only be considered if there is evidence of cervical change with intact membranes. Uterine rupture is associated with extremely high rates of fetal mortality. Placental abruption may occur up to 48 hours after the accident and close monitoring of mother and fetus is necessary. The first sign may be that of fetal compromise and the abdomen will be tense. Amniotic fluid embolism may also occur.

Feto-maternal Haemorrhage: If rhesus positive fetal blood cells gain access to the circulation of a rhesus positive mother she may become sensitized, compromising subsequent pregnancies unless she receives a sufficient dose of Anti D. The Kleihauer-Betke blood test can ascertain the amount of fetal cells in a maternal blood sample indicating the magnitude of fetal haemorrhage and allowing precise titration of Anti D treatment.

15.6.3 **Assessment**

15.6.3.1 *The primary survey*

This deals with immediate life-threatening injuries according to a standardized A and Cervical Spine, B, C approach, plus prompt relief of aortocaval compression:

- A = Airway (C Spine): Clear and open airway, immobilising the cervical spine if indicated. Use airway adjuncts and deliver the highest concentration oxygen possible using artificial ventilation if necessary. Consider intubation with cricoid pressure and anticipate difficulties with relation to position and the anatomical changes of pregnancy
- B = Breathing: Identify and treat major thoracic injuries:
- Pneumothorax—insert large bore cannula into the 2nd intercostal space in the mid-clavicular line, followed by a chest drain
- Haemopneumothorax—as above but ensure large bore (28F and above). Thoracotomy will be required if blood loss is > 1500 ml.
- C = Circulation and Haemorrhage Control. Relieve aortocaval compression to optimize cardiac output. Establish two large bore intravenous cannulae and take blood for cross matching, full blood count, urea, and electrolytes and clotting screen. Compress obvious bleeding points. Do not place packs in the vagina if there is vaginal bleeding. Start a rapid infusion of warmed crystalloid solution (2–3 ml/kg) and assess response. Aim to maintain vital organ perfusion without elevating systolic pressures too high, which can increase further bleeding.

15.6.3.2 *Secondary survey*

This is the 'top to toe' examination and may include re-assessment of the primary survey. It is only performed after the primary survey and treatment and stabilization of life threatening injuries.

15.6.4 **Imaging**

X-ray images of the cervical spine, chest, and pelvis should be taken as soon as the patient is stabilized and should not be deferred because of pregnancy.

Chapter 16

Pre-eclampsia

Rachel Collis

Key points

- Pre-eclampsia can rapidly result in the death of mother and baby
- It can be diagnosed early by regular measurement of the mother's blood pressure and testing her urine for protein
- A blood pressure above 140/90 mmHg and 2+ proteinuria are important indicators of the diagnosis
- The severity of hypertension or proteinurea does not correlate with the severity of the disease
- Death results from eclampsia, cerebral haemorrhage, hepatic rupture, renal failure, or pulmonary oedema causing respiratory failure
- Early delivery of the baby will stop progression of the condition and save the mother's life.

16.1 Classification and diagnosis

Pre-eclampsia (PET) is a multi-system disorder occurring exclusively after the 20th week of pregnancy and affects up to 8% of all pregnancies. It is one diagnosis that forms part of the spectrum of hypertensive disorders of pregnancy. It can be separate from other hypertensive disorders or overlap with them, as some women with other causes of hypertension are much more likely to develop pre-eclampsia. Hypertension in pregnancy is defined as a manual BP reading >140 mmHg systolic and/or >90 mmHg diastolic (using Korotkoff Phase V) on two consecutive occasions more than 4 hours apart or one blood pressure of 110 mmHg diastolic or more. Most automated blood pressure monitors under-estimate blood pressure and a high index of suspicion should lead to manual checking with an appropriate size cuff. Pre-existing hypertension causes the blood pressure to be raised earlier in the pregnancy, is not usually associated with proteinurea, but can worsen hypertension in later pregnancy. The diagnosis of proteinurea is made by urine dip stick of

2+ on two consecutive occasions in the absence of a urinary infection or > 300mg/24hour urine collection.

16.1.1 **Risk factors**

Any woman can develop pre-eclampsia, although a number of risk factors make it more likely. These include; first pregnancy or more than 10 years since the last pregnancy, a new partner, a previous history of pre-eclampsia, a first degree female family relative with the disease, maternal age > 40yr, obesity, multiple pregnancy and other medical conditions such as renal disease or diabetes.

16.1.2 **Other features of the diagnosis**

The three features of increased blood pressure, proteinurea and peripheral oedema are important in the diagnosis, but they may be mild and the underlying disease severe. Pre-eclampsia may cause severe intra-uterine growth restriction of the fetus leading to fetal death with few other signs. HELLP syndrome which is a severe form of pre-eclampsia, i.e. **H**aemolytic anaemia, **E**levated **L**iver enzymes and **L**ow **P**latelets can present with a normal blood pressure but these complications can lead to maternal death if not rapidly diagnosed and treated.

16.1.3 **Pathophysiology of pre-eclampsia**

The exact cause of pre-eclampsia is not known but it is thought to be a widespread problem of endothelial cell dysfunction within blood vessels throughout the body. It is thought that the placenta develops abnormally during the first few weeks of gestation which predisposes to pre-eclampsia later on.

16.1.3.1 Cardiovascular changes

There is generalized vasoconstriction in all blood vessels. This leads to an increase in systemic vascular resistance (SVR) and hypertension. The capillaries become more permeable and as a result, fluid leaks into the interstitial space causing oedema. In severe cases, pulmonary and cerebral oedema can be life threatening.

16.1.3.2 Respiratory changes

Pulmonary oedema causes the mother's oxygen saturation to decrease and the work of breathing to increase. She may be breathless with rapid shallow breathing. Oedema around the face and neck can make intubation during general anaesthesia difficult. A husky voice can be an early sign of oedema of the vocal cords.

16.1.3.3 Renal changes

Damage to the endothelial lining of the blood vessels of the kidneys causes proteinurea initially, but eventually can lead to acute renal failure. A raised uric acid can be an early marker and a high normal creatinine and urea may be significant.

16.1.3.4 Hepatic changes

Liver distension causing epigastic pain and occasionally liver rupture, along with rapidly rising AST, ALT and gamma GT can be part of pre-eclampsia. It is usually associated with HELLP syndrome, but can present without haemolytic anaemia and low platelets and only mildly elevated blood pressure.

16.1.3.5 Central nervous system

Cerebral oedema and vasoconstriction may cause eclamptic seizures. Although often associated with raised blood pressure, this is not always the case. High blood pressure is usually the direct cause of cerebral haemorrhage but may be transitory. Headache, vomiting, confusion, hyper-reflexia and clonus are all part of the syndrome.

16.1.3.6 Haematological changes

Low platelets and anaemia associated with haemolysis is usually associated with HELLP syndrome but can occur alone with raised blood pressure. Abnormal blood clotting is only associated with significantly deranged liver function.

16.1.3.7 Feto-placental unit

Severe intra-uterine growth restriction is often seen and may be evident many weeks before the mother develops raised blood pressure and the other signs of pre-eclampsia. There is significant risk of placental abruption and severe haemorrhage. In other cases, fetal death from growth restriction may be the only obvious sign of pre-eclampsia.

16.2 Antenatal management of PET

If hypertension and proteinuria are both mild and there are no other signs of pre-eclampsia as outlined above, pregnancy may be prolonged to allow fetal maturation using oral anti-hypertensive drugs. Methyldopa has a long safety record in pregnancy, labetalol is safe for the mother but can cause neonatal hypoglycaemia after the baby is born, and nifedipine is especially beneficial for short term, rapid blood pressure control. There is no evidence that one is better than the other. Anti-hypertensives that should be avoided are other beta-blockers, diuretics and ACE inhibitors. There is good evidence that good blood pressure control can reduce the incidence of severe pre-eclampsia by 50%, but it is important to remember that blood pressure control does not cure pre-eclampsia, only delivery will do that. The mother and baby should be regularly monitored 2 or 3 times per week to ensure that severe problems are not developing.

16.2.1 Severe pre-eclampsia

Around 5/1000 pregnancies are complicated by severe pre-eclampsia that can be life threatening for the mother and baby. It is also important to remember that it is possible to have severe pre-eclampsia with normal or mildly raised blood pressure. Pre-eclampsia can be defined as severe if two blood pressure readings are > 170 systolic and/or 110 diastolic 4 hours apart with proteinuria >1gram/L or 3+++ on dip stick OR more moderately raised blood pressure 140/90 with 2++ proteinuria and any two from the following list: severe headache, visual disturbance, clonus (3 or more beats) papilloedema, epigastric pain, platelets <100x10^9 or abnormal LFTs.

16.2.2 Eclampsia

Eclampsia is one or more generalized convulsions superimposed on any degree of pre-eclampsia. It affects 5 in 10,000 pregnancies and is associated with at least 2% mortality, although this may be considerably higher if not promptly treated. Although more eclamptic seizures occur antenatally, around 30% occur post natally and up to several days post delivery.

16.2.3 Management of severe pre-eclampsia

The mother should be admitted to hospital, if possible, as she will probably need to be delivered within the next 24–48 hours. She should have her blood pressure measured and recorded at least every hour and blood tests for haemoglobin, platelet count, renal function and liver function requested if available. The baby should be monitored because fetal distress and demise is common. Blood pressure can be controlled with oral drugs as above, but if hypertension is severe, intravenous labetalol or hydralazine are more effective. 50mg labetalol IV should be given over 10 minutes followed by an infusion to a maximum of 480mg/hr. IV hydralazine 5mg over 20 minutes is more effective but can occasionally dramatically reduce blood pressure. It should be given with IV fluids and the mother's blood pressure monitored every 5 minutes. Oral nifedipine 10–20mg can be given but may have a synergistic action with magnesium; therefore, close monitoring is required. Magnesium given IM or IV reduces the risk of an eclamptic fit in severe pre-eclampsia and is now frequently combined with anti-hypertensives. It reduces the fluctuations in blood pressure and ensures greater blood pressure stability, with reduced requirements for additional anti-hypertensives. However, magnesium should not replace the use of effective anti-hypertensives.

16.2.4 Timing and mode of delivery

To improve the mother's chance of survival, she may need to be delivered severely prematurely, i.e. before 34 weeks gestation. Oral steriods given 24 hours prior to delivery are safe in pre-eclampsia and may improve the outlook of a premature baby even if neonatal intensive care is not available. After 34 weeks gestation, survival of the baby improves and delivery can be by caesarean section or vaginal birth depending on facilities and how quickly delivery is required.

16.3 **Fluid balance**

16.3.1 **General principles (see Figure 16.1)**

Excessive fluid administration is harmful to the mother in severe pre-eclampsia as it increases the risk of pulmonary and cerebral oedema. Restricting oral or intravenous fluid intake to 1 ml/kg/hr is safe. Fluid restriction should start when the diagnosis of severe pre-eclampsia is made, and should be continued until after the delivery of the baby when spontaneous diuresis occurs. This is usually in the first 24 hours. Recording the mother's fluid input and her urine output is important. A urine output of >0.5 ml/kg/hr is satisfactory. A pulse

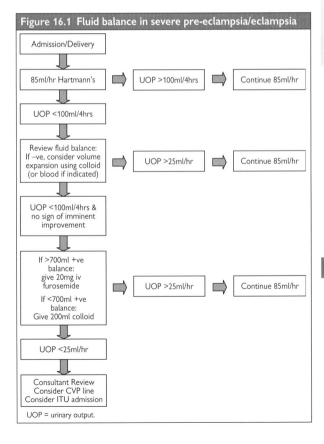

Figure 16.1 Fluid balance in severe pre-eclampsia/eclampsia

Admission/Delivery

→ 85ml/hr Hartmann's ⇒ UOP >100ml/4hrs ⇒ Continue 85ml/hr

→ UOP <100ml/4hrs

→ Review fluid balance: If −ve, consider volume expansion using colloid (or blood if indicated) ⇒ UOP >25ml/hr ⇒ Continue 85ml/hr

→ UOP <100ml/4hrs & no sign of imminent improvement

→ If >700ml +ve balance: give 20mg iv furosemide

If <700ml +ve balance: Give 200ml colloid ⇒ UOP >25ml/hr ⇒ Continue 85ml/hr

→ UOP <25ml/hr

→ Consultant Review Consider CVP line Consider ITU admission

UOP = urinary output.

131

oximeter is extremely useful if available. Decreasing oxygen saturations are an early sign of pulmonary oedema (<94% on air), although counting the mother's respiratory rate is also helpful (RR>25/min). Although acute renal failure can occur with severe pre-eclampsia, it is nearly always associated with concurrent haemorrhage rather than moderate fluid restriction as described above.

16.3.2 Diuretic administration

The administration of a diuretic drug will not alter the disease or reduce the risk of acute renal failure. A diuresis is commonly seen following IV furosemide, therefore it can be useful in the management of a positive fluid balance of >1500-2000 ml over a 24 hour period, where there is a risk or actual diagnosis of pulmonary oedema.

16.4 Eclampsia

16.4.1 Prevention

The MAGPIE trial showed that use of IV magnesium sulphate reduced a mother's risk of having an eclamptic fit by 58%. It is most commonly administered to severe pre-eclamptic women, if there is a family or personal history of eclampsia or if there are prominent neurological symptoms such as clonus or confusion.

Magnesium loading dose
For those women not on magnesium sulphate already **Administer 4 grams IV over 5 minutes** Draw up 10 ml of 50% magnesium sulphate (5 gm) with 40 ml normal saline, to give a total volume of 50 ml. Give 40 ml over 5–10 minutes. For those already on an infusion of magnesium sulphate Take blood for urgent Mg^{2+} level and **give additional 2 gm IV** (20 ml of above mixture) over 10 minutes.

16.4.2 Treatment of eclampsia

The mother should be placed in the full left lateral position and her **A**irway, **B**reathing and **C**irculation assessed and supported. Oxygen should be administered by face mask. An IV line should be inserted and IV magnesium administered, as described above. If blood testing is available, FBC, clotting screen, U&Es and LFTs should be done.

If an IV line is **NOT** available, 4 gm of magnesium sulphate can be injected IM into a large muscle mass e.g. buttock area. Monitoring of ECG, blood pressure and oxygen saturation is beneficial. Most fits associated with eclampsia are short-lived and self-terminating. Magnesium will terminate a fit and it is safer than other anti-convulsant drugs e.g. diazepam or other benzodiazepines. Magnesium must be given with caution in hepatic coma, renal failure, myasthenia gravis, absent or diminished tendon reflexes and if nifedipine has been given.

After administration of a magnesium loading dose, an infusion should be started to reduce the risk of a further eclamptic fit:

Magnesium maintenance infusion

1 gm/hr
Dilute 30 ml of 50% magnesium sulphate with 30 ml of N.Saline = 60ml x 25% $MgSO_4$ (0.25 gm/ml) – infuse at 4 ml/hour

---

The usual doses of magnesium should be reduced, e.g. typically halved, in the presence of significant renal dysfunction, e.g. urine output < 100 ml/4 hrs or an elevated urea or creatinine level.

16.4.3 **Complications of eclampsia**

Failure to recover consciousness or recurrent convulsions are an indication for intubation and immediate caesarean delivery. Fetal distress is also very common. If there is no fetal distress and the seizures are controlled, it is best practice to stabilize the mother's blood pressure before delivery.

16.4.4 **Magnesium therapy**

If given in excessive doses or if the mother has renal failure, magnesium can produce toxicity. Early signs are muscle weakness, respiratory depression, and absent tendon reflexes. Severe toxicity will result in muscle paralysis, respiratory arrest, heart block, and cardiac arrest. Routine monitoring of magnesium levels is not considered necessary, although if toxicity is suspected, they may be useful. If severe toxicity is suspected, treatment must not be delayed whilst waiting for blood results.

Treatment of suspected magnesium toxicity

Absent tendon reflexes and respiratory rate <14/min

- Stop magnesium infusion
- Support respiratory/cardiovascular systems as per ALS algorithm
- Calcium gluconate 1 gm (10ml) over 10 minutes should be given for signs of significant toxicity.

The infusion should be restarted at half the previous rate once respiratory depression has resolved.

Magnesium affects the neuromuscular junction and increases the effect of depolarizing muscle relaxants, and reduces the appearance of fasciculations, but not the effect, of suxamethonium. It also causes vasodilatation, which may potentiate the effect of other anti-hypertensives. It also causes a minor inhibition of uterine contractions.

16.5 Anaesthetic management of the mother with pre-eclampsia

16.5.1 Labour

Many women over 37 weeks gestation can labour safely with a diagnosis of pre-eclampsia, provided their blood pressure is well controlled and the condition not rapidly worsening.

16.5.1.1 Epidural analgesia

If available, epidural analgesia is ideal because blood pressure control is improved. A platelet count taken in the previous 4 hours should be available and above 80×10^9 before the epidural sited. Usual epidural precautions should then be employed.

16.5.2 Caesarean section

Ideally, the patient should be fully pre-assessed, fasted and have received antacid prophylaxis. The mother's blood pressure should be controlled and recent blood tests available. If her condition is very unstable, this may not be possible. Blood pressure monitoring during the operation is required and oxygen saturation preferable. A wide-bore IV cannula should be inserted, with fluids available in case of haemorrhage. After the operation the mother should NOT receive non-steroidal anti-inflammatory drugs for postoperative pain relief, until she passes adequate volume of urine i.e. >100ml/hr.

16.5.2.1 Regional anaesthesia

A regional technique is preferable to a general anaesthetic and can usually be safely performed. The mother must, however, be conscious, cooperative and preferably have a platelet count above 80. Pre-load should be minimal and fluids are not usually required to control hypotension. Prophylactic vasopressors should not be used, and if the mother becomes hypotensive (systolic BP <100 mmHg), only small doses of a vasopressor should be given because of an increased sensitivity leading to rebound hypertension.

The easiest technique is spinal anaesthesia, although an epidural top-up or combined spinal epidural technique can be performed. It was thought for many years that a spinal anaesthetic was dangerous because of sudden severe hypotension. This does not seem to be the case in practice and with the usual simple precautions, it is a rapid, safe and effective technique. A standard dose of local anaesthetic with an opiate, if available, should be used.

16.5.2.2 General anaesthesia

A general anaesthetic may be required if immediate delivery is required, if convulsions are poorly controlled, in event of severe hemorrhage, if the low platelet count is <80 or clotting screen abnormal. However, a general anaesthetic is associated with greater risks than a spinal anaesthetic. Facial and laryngeal oedema can make intubation extremely difficult, pulmonary oedema can make oxygenation impossible and the blood pressure surges associated with intubation and extubation can lead to cerebral haemorrhage.

Careful airway assessment is essential. Voice changes, hoarseness and stridor will alert the anaesthetist to the possibility of laryngeal oedema. Pre-operative administration of 0.2mg/kg dexamethasone IV can be helpful. A smaller tracheal tube than usual may be necessary and should be available down to a size 6mm.

The blood pressure should be monitored regularly during induction, maintenance and emergence of anaesthesia. The blood pressure response to intubation can be obtunded with a short acting IV opiate such as fentanyl 100–200mcg or alfentanil 1–2mg, IV labetalol 50–100mg or 2–4 gram of IV magnesium. The dose of magnesium will depend on the size of the patient and whether magnesium has already been given. A small patient should have the dose reduced from 2 to 1 gram and a large patient from 4 to 2 grams.

Thiopental 3–5mg/Kg should be given, as light anaesthesia at induction will make hypertensive surges worse. Ketamine should be avoided if possible. The short acting muscle relaxant suxamethonium will facilitate rapid intubation, but if magnesium has been given, the usual fasciculations will be less prominent, although muscle relaxation will be unaffected. A balanced anaesthetic technique with oxygen, nitrous oxide, volatile agents, and opiates should be used if possible. If magnesium has been used, a smaller dose of any long acting muscle relaxant should be given (reduce by 25%), as magnesium potentiates the non-depolarizing effect. Neostigmine with atropine or glycopyrronium and monitoring of neuromuscluar function is preferable prior to extubation. Large surges in blood pressure can also be caused by extubation; close monitoring is required and additional doses of antihypertensives or magnesium may be needed. It is very common for the mother to become normotensive or mildly hypotensive during general anaesthesia, but regular monitoring of blood pressure should be continued into the postoperative period as hypertension will frequently become problematic again.

16.5.3 **Post delivery management**

Regardless of the mode of delivery, the mother should be closely monitored for at least 24 hours as complications can continue to be problematic. Severe hypertension can cause cerebral hemorrhage and 30% of eclamptic fits occur after delivery. Fluids should be restricted to about 80 ml/hr until a natural post delivery diuresis occurs. Morphine and paracetamol can safely be given if the mother has had a caesarean section, but NSAIDs should be avoided. If the mother is on a magnesium infusion, it should ideally be continued for 24 hours post delivery or a second IM dose of magnesium administered. Oral anti-hypertensives can usually replace intravenous drugs within this time period.

Chapter 17

Obstetric haemorrhage

Sue Catling

Key points

- Major haemorrhage is defined as a single blood loss of >1500 ml, continuing blood loss of 150 ml/hr or a transfusion requirement of 4 units of red cells
- The early team approach to managing major haemorrhage will improve the outcome for the mother
- Early resuscitation is essential
- Early diagnosis of the cause of major haemorrhage will focus therapy and can be easily remembered by thinking of the 4Ts
- Specialist techniques of balloon tamponade or B-Lynch suture are effective in persistent uterine atony
- Coagulation failure occurs early in obstetric haemorrhage and should be corrected if possible
- Aftercare of the mother with regular monitoring of heart rate, blood pressure, urine output will improve outcome.

17.1 Organizational aspects of managing major obstetric haemorrhage

17.1.1 Prevention and planning

It is important to try to identify the patient at risk of major haemorrhage by understanding the known risk factors which include; grand multi-parity, increased maternal age, multiple pregnancy, women with complex medical problems, prolonged and/or obstructed labour and where there is placental abruption or fetal death.

Beware of the patient who has had a previous CS and presents with a placenta praevia in her current pregnancy. She is at high risk of placenta accreta, a condition where the placenta grows into the previous scar tissue. The placenta does not separate after delivery, the uterus cannot contract and life threatening haemorrhage rapidly follows. These patients should only be delivered, if at all possible, where blood transfusion facilities exist.

17.1.2 Preparation (practice, protocols and audit)

A team approach between obstetricians, anaesthetists, midwives, and theatre staff is essential, including good communication and effective action. Without team skills, the patient may still die despite individual clinical skill and effort. Communication and team building exercises or drills can be organized outside clinical time and have been shown to reduce the number of deaths. Written local protocols, to which every member of the team has contributed and are specifically designed to work in the local environment, are beneficial. If problems arise during the management of major haemorrhage, time should be made afterwards for discussion so that improvements can be made for future events.

17.2 Clinical management

17.2.1 Overview

The aim of management is to rapidly restore circulating volume and prevent tissue hypoxia. Initial resuscitation will be the same whatever the cause of the haemorrhage. Subsequent obstetric management will depend on whether the baby is delivered and/or viable. In many cases, the patient will require an anaesthetic for exploration of the uterus and surgical haemostasis. During on-going, severe haemorrhage, senior anaesthetic and obstetric help should be sought if available. A blood transfusion will usually be required once the blood loss exceeds 2500ml and blood bank and haematology services will need to be alerted. The operating obstetrician should be confident that she/he can perform a caesarean hysterectomy.

17.2.2 Role of the anaesthetist

The anaesthetist can initiate and lead the resuscitation and stabilization, including the estimation of blood loss and appropriate ordering of blood and blood products. The anaesthetist has responsibility to administer an appropriate anaesthetic technique to allow surgical exploration, administer drugs to control haemorrhage and appropriate fluid replacement, set up monitoring and help organize appropriate postoperative critical care.

17.2.3 Initial resuscitation and stabilization

Any resuscitation should follow the obstetric ABC principle as follows:
• Tilt—if still pregnant
• 100% Oxygen
• ABC with rapid initial assessment and correction as found
• Diagnosis and Definitive treatment.

17.2.3.1 Tilt

Prior to delivery, supine aorto-caval compression must be avoided by placing the patient in either the left lateral position or providing 15 degrees left lateral tilt with a wedge under the right hip. If the patient is supine, the gravid uterus will compress the vena cava and prevent adequate venous return to the heart. This will reduce cardiac output by up to 30%, worsening hypotension due to blood loss and prevent effective resuscitation. If neither manoeuvre is possible, the uterus must be manually displaced to the left.

17.2.3.2 Oxygen

Administer 15 litres/minute oxygen or as much as is available, via a tight-fitting face mask with a reservoir bag if possible. This will achieve optimal oxygen saturation of the blood remaining in the circulation and help to prevent tissue hypoxia. In addition, the nitrogen in the functional residual capacity of the lungs will be washed out and replaced by oxygen—this provides a valuable reservoir for continuing oxygenation of pulmonary blood should respiratory compromise occur.

17.2.3.3 Airway

A severely shocked patient may lose consciousness due to hypotension and require tracheal intubation to protect the airway from gastric acid aspiration and to maintain adequate oxygenation/ventilation.

17.2.3.4 Breathing

This may become inadequate and the patient may require ventilation as consciousness is lost and as severe tissue hypoxia and metabolic acidosis supervene.

17.2.3.5 Circulation

Rapid assessment of the estimated blood volume lost should be done at the same time as 2 x wide bore (14G) IV cannulae are inserted, basic monitoring applied if available i.e. pulse oximeter, non-invasive blood pressure, ECG, but **do not delay fluid resuscitation**—the pulse rate, pulse volume and capillary refill time are reliable indicators of hypovolaemia.

When blood loss is estimated to be less than 30% of the blood volume (up to 2000 ml), IV crystalloid or colloid fluid resuscitation may be adequate. However, when blood loss has reached 50% of blood volume, the mother will almost certainly require a blood transfusion.

Once the diagnosis of major haemorrhage has been made, take 20ml blood for FBC, coagulation screen and cross match blood, if possible.

Common pitfall: Normal blood pressure does not exclude major blood loss in the pregnant patient

The physiologically increased plasma volume and red cell mass in pregnancy means total blood volume is increased up to 40%. Therefore, up to 40% blood volume can be lost (1500–2000 ml) before any degree of hypotension is apparent. This is because blood is shunted away from the feto-placental unit (750 ml/minute) to maintain flow to vital organs such as the brain, heart, and kidneys.

Early signs of impending maternal collapse with a normal blood pressure include:

- Tachycardia >100 bpm
- Fetal distress
- Skin pallor with increased capillary refill time (>2 seconds, or the time it takes to say 'capillary refill')
- Decreased/absent urine output <30 ml/hr, this is often not apparent in the acute situation.

Signs of life-threatening hypovolaemia i.e. > 50% blood volume loss include:

- Hypotension
- Tachypnoea
- Mental clouding, progressing to unconsciousness.

Ensure that all blood sampling is correctly labelled and inform blood bank of the degree of urgency. It is often useful to delegate a team member to this task, and also to assign someone to record all events, with timings.

Infuse 2 L of crystalloid (Hartmanns/Normal Saline) rapidly and set up a blood warming device and pressure infuser, if available. The patient may need to be transferred to theatre at the same time, and the obstetrician should establish the underlying cause of bleeding and decide on the surgical management plan.

Assess the response to initial volume replacement:

- 15–30% blood loss (750–1500 ml) will respond to crystalloids alone; tachycardia will improve and remain improved
- 30–40% blood loss (1500–2000 ml) will have a transitory response to crystalloids and will require colloid infusion while waiting for cross matched or group specific blood
- >50% blood loss (>2500 ml) is life-threatening and requires blood transfusion as soon as possible.

17.2.4 **Monitoring**

The mother will require regular heart rate and blood pressure monitoring. During active bleeding, this should be at 5-minute intervals. If bleeding is extreme, direct arterial monitoring and/or CVP monitoring can provide additional measurements to aid the management of fluid replacement. These additional techniques should only be used if readily available and there is experience with their use because insertion can be difficult and cause significant harm. Urine output is a simple and useful guide to successful fluid management. After major blood loss, it may take several hours for normal urine output to be restored (>30 ml/hr) even with adequate fluid management. An indwelling urinary catheter will help monitoring. Oxygen saturation gives beat to beat assessment of adequate oxygenation and should be used if possible. It is also a useful aid in the diagnosis of pulmonary oedema, which is common after major blood loss and rapid fluid replacement.

17.3 **The 4Ts: Directed therapy and definitive treatment**

The classic causes of antepartum obstetric haemorrhage are ruptured ectopic pregnancy, placenta praevia, placental abruption, vasa praevia, and uterine rupture. During the postpartum period, haemorrhage may be due to uterine atony, retained uterine products, unrecognized ongoing surgical bleeding, uterine inversion, vaginal lacerations, or placenta accreta. There must be a logical and step wise approach to the diagnosis, so that effective drug and surgical therapy can be initiated. In order to establish the cause of bleeding, the lower genital tract should be examined for tears or lacerations and the uterus and pelvis should be explored if retained products, uterine rupture or uncontrolled surgical bleeding are suspected or uterine atony persists. When the underlying cause has been established, a definitive treatment plan can be made, e.g. additional uterotonic drugs, surgery for lacerations or if continued bleeding after caesarean section, uterine tamponade techniques or a hysterectomy may be performed.

A practical, working classification of the causes of major obstetric haemorrhage is to use the classification of **The 4Ts: Tone, Tissue, Trauma or Thrombin?**

17.3.1 **'Tone'**

17.3.1.1 Mechanical

The simple 'rubbing-up' of a contraction is an effective skill, which should be used early. Placing a hand on the abdomen and firmly rubbing the fundus of the uterus. Bimanual compression (compressing the fundus and base of uterus together between two hands) can be used at vaginal or operative delivery and may be a life saving initial measure.

17.3.1.2 Drugs

The routine administration of uterotonic drugs at delivery can dramatically reduce the risk of haemorrhage due to uterine atony. The usual first choice of drug is oxytocin or a mixture of oxytocin and ergometrine given IM or IV. Oxytocin, ergomentrine, carboprost and misoprostal are all effective and any can be used in a stepwise fashion or singularly, if only one is available, once uterine atony has been diagnosed.

Oxytocin should be given as a slow IV bolus of 5 IU, followed by an IV infusion of 40 IU over 4 hours diluted in saline in the event of anticipated or ongoing postpartum haemorrhage.

Ergometrine 0.5 mg IM or IV causes uterine and vascular smooth muscle contraction through 5-HT receptor stimulation. It should be used with extreme caution in pre-eclampsia and heart disease.

Misoprostol is a synthetic PGE1 prostaglandin analogue that increases uterine tone. It is administered rectally in a dose of 600–1000mcg and is very effective, easy to store and relatively inexpensive.

Carboprost (15-methyl PGF2) is a potent synthetic analogue of prostaglandin (PG) F2 alpha, which is given IM (or intra-myometrially) in doses of 250mcg. It can be repeated every 15 minutes to a maximum total dose of 2 mg. Carboprost can cause hypoxia due to intrapulmonary shunting caused by pulmonary vascular smooth muscle constriction. It should NOT be given IV and should be used with caution in pre-eclampsia or heart disease.

Prostaglandins PGE1 and PGF2 stimulate myometrial contraction and should be considered if oxytocics or ergometrine fail to achieve adequate myometrial contraction.

17.3.2 'Tissue'

The uterus must be empty for effective contraction to occur, therefore any remaining fragments of placenta, blood clot or membranes must be removed. This can sometimes be done gently after a vaginal delivery without anaesthesia, but frequently requires more detailed investigation and adequate anaesthesia. An abnormally adherent or invasive placenta, e.g. accreta can pose particular problems necessitating hysterectomy.

17.3.3 'Trauma'

Lacerations and tears to the uterus or lower genital tract are a common and frequently under-estimated cause of hemorrhage. They must be carefully explored and repaired under anaesthesia. General anaesthesia will usually be required if bleeding is ongoing or there is any degree of haemodynamic instability. Regional anaesthesia should only be considered if the patient is fully resuscitated, haemodynamically stable and has satisfactory clotting.

17.3.4 'Thrombin'

Initial fluid resuscitation is based on volume replacement and clinical assessment. The Hb level is often a poor indicator of blood loss in acute bleeding. It has been shown in clinical reconstruction scenarios that blood loss is **underestimated by up to 35%** by most clinical groups. If possible, an FBC to assess Hb and platelet count, and clotting screen should be taken for laboratory assessment. Once coagulation failure has occurred, it is very difficult to stop obstetric haemorrhage by drug or surgical therapy alone.

17.4 Blood transfusion and clotting factors

17.4.1 Red cell transfusion

If blood loss is 50% or greater than the blood volume (>2500 ml), whole blood or packed red cells in an additive solution should be transfused. Aim for a Hb level of 8.0 g/dl; over-transfusion is unnecessary. **O Negative** blood can be used in an extreme emergency. **Fully cross matched** blood is preferable if time allows.

17.4.2 Platelets

The platelet count needs to be maintained above 50×10^9/L if haemorrhage is on-going. A fall to this level is typical of a 2 blood volume replacement, or less if there is associated disseminated intravascular coagulation (DIC). An ideal dose of platelets for transfusion is 1 adult therapeutic dose for every 4 units of transfused red cells. Very low platelet counts are associated with placental abruption—early recognition and aggressive treatment is required.

17.4.3 FFP and cryoprecipitate

Coagulation failure is common in major obstetric haemorrhage. The onset can be very rapid when haemorrhage is caused by antenatal abruption leading to DIC. Coagulation failure is also caused by giving large quantities of crystalloid, colloid, or stored blood that do not contain clotting factors. This leads to dilutional coagulation failure. The ideal combination is to give 4 units of fresh frozen plasma (FFP) with every 4 units of red cells transfused, if there is ongoing bleeding. FFP can be given on clinical grounds alone with rapid blood loss or after checking a clotting screen. FFP contains all the coagulation factors but is a relatively poor source of fibrinogen. Cryoprecipitate is relatively poor in some of the clotting factors but has more fibrinogen. Normothermia is essential for haemostasis, therefore use of IV fluid warmers and surface warming devices are essential.

17.4.4 **Antifibrinolytics: drugs to inhibit clot lysis**

Tranexamic acid is an anti-fibrinolytic agent, which competitively inhibits the conversion of plasminogen to plasmin, thereby preventing fibrin degradation and stabilizing clot formation. It can be given by slow IV injection at a dose of 0.5–1.0 gm and it can be given with other blood products.

17.5 **Specialist techniques**

If the uterus remains atonic and bleeding continues despite giving appropriate uterotonics and removal of possible retained products, specialist surgical techniques are necessary. The early use of physical methods to control on-going bleeding is changing the management of major obstetric hemorrhage and reduces the side effects associated with the over use of uterotonics. **A hysterectomy** has been considered the definitive life-saving treatment for haemorrhage, and whilst this may still be appropriate in some cases, effective alternatives are now available with which the anaesthetist needs to be familiar.

17.5.1 **Balloon tamponade of uterus**

Hydrostatic balloons can be used within the uterine cavity to control haemorrhage, both for atony and placenta accreta. The Rusch Balloon can be inflated with 600ml of saline and left in situ for 48hrs, then gradually deflated over several hours. A Senstaken balloon for oesophageal varices and even a condom tied over a urinary catheter and inflated with saline have been used with success in this situation. The uterus can also be packed with gauze, but this requires a more traumatic removal.

17.5.2 **B-Lynch brace suture**

This is a surgical technique of 'folding' the atonic uterus down on itself to provide compression haemostasis (Figure 17.1). In the UK Report into Confidential Enquiries into Maternal and Child Health (CEMACH) 2000–2002, there were **no deaths** in patients in whom this had been used. The use of the B-Lynch suture can avoid the need for hysterectomy, and there are reports of successful pregnancies after its use.

17.5.3 **Transfusion alternatives—cell salvage**

Where access to a safe blood supply is not possible, this specialist technique for washing, concentrating and returning the patient's own blood can provide a useful source of red blood cells. It also reduces the patient's exposure to donor blood and conserves the blood supply in massive bleeding. It is now being used widely in the UK and USA. If blood is salvaged in this way, it does not contain clotting factors, so they will need to be given in addition.

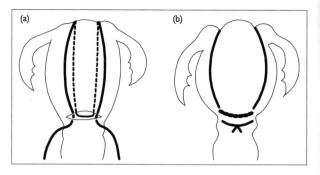

Figure 17.1 B-Lynch suture. (a) A single suture is inserted as shown. (b) As it is drawn tight, the fundus of the uterus is compressed against the lower segment. The uterus is now physically unable to relax.

17.6 **Anaesthesia**

The choice of anaesthetic technique must be left to the individual skill and experience of the anaesthetist. However, as a general principle, if the mother does not already have a regional anaesthetic in-situ, consider a GA if haemorrhage is severe, there is on-going haemodynamic instability or the diagnosis is uncertain. If there is a spinal or epidural in situ, surgery may continue safely, as conversion to general anaethesia may make the haemodynamic instability worse. There are many case reports of caesarean hysterectomies performed solely under regional techniques. A regional technique should be converted to GA if the woman becomes unconsciousness due to hypotension or has inadequate anaesthesia, especially during prolonged surgery.

17.7 **Continuing care and lessons learned**

Following major obstetric haemorrhage, the mother must be carefully monitored in an appropriate safe environment. Maternal deaths have been attributed to sub-standard care in the postpartum period. All mothers where the bleeding has been estimated > 1500 ml are best cared for in a high dependency environment, even if apparently stable. Hourly observations should be made of pulse rate, blood pressure, urine output, respiratory rate and fluid balance, especially in the first 6 hours. Regular Hb and coagulation studies will need to be performed every 4–6 hours, if the blood transfusion requirements are >8 units.

Postoperative ventilation is indicated if there is on-going bleeding, especially if associated with uncorrected clotting abnormalities, hypothermia, severe oliguria/anuria, pulmonary oedema and poorly corrected metabolic acidosis with an increased lactate >2.0.

17.7.1 **Review**

All staff involved in cases of major obstetric haemorrhage should conduct a 'rapid review' of the case, ideally within 48 hours, to examine the effectiveness of the systems involved, to define the lessons learnt and to organize support and counselling as necessary in the event of a bad outcome.

Chapter 18

Embolic disease

Raman Sivasankar, Sarah Harries

Key points

- Women are 2–5 times more likely to develop a deep vein thrombosis or suffer a pulmonary embolism during or immediately after pregnancy
- Malaria and sickle cell disease are additional risk factors
- Clinical suspicion of thrombo-embolism should be investigated further and treated with a safe anticoagulant regimen during pregnancy and for at least 6 weeks postpartum
- Subcutaneous heparin injection is the mainstay of treatment antenatally, whilst warfarin may be used postpartum
- Delivery should be planned in advance when a woman is receiving anticoagulant treatment as she is at significant risk of bleeding
- Regional anaesthetic techniques are contra-indicated if the clotting screen is abnormal
- Thrombo-prophylaxis should be given to all mothers following caesarean section according to body weight
- Amniotic fluid embolism and massive air embolism are rare complications of delivery.

18.1 Venous thrombo-embolism (VTE)

VTE is an important cause of morbidity and mortality in pregnant women and is a leading cause of maternal death. Pregnant women are 2 to 5 times more likely to develop VTE compared to non-pregnant women. Two thirds of deep vein thromboses occur in the antepartum period; however, the postpartum period carries the highest risk.

18.1.1 Risk factors for VTE in pregnancy

Recognized risk factors include: concurrent infection, sickle cell disease, malaria, personal or family history of VTE, obesity, age >35 years, smoking, pre-eclampsia, postpartum haemorrhage, caesarean section, diabetes, and thrombophilia.

Malaria increases coagulability by causing a cytokine storm in the host in response to the infection, which promotes thrombosis. The activation of the monocyte-macrophage system also has a part to play, as do the drugs used to treat malaria. Sickle cell disease and its variants can also be a cause of thrombo-embolism. An acute chest syndrome associated with these conditions presents with an acute episode of fever, chest pain and dyspnoea and may mimic a pulmonary embolism.

18.1.2 Pathophysiology

The triad responsible for VTE in pregnancy includes altered coagulation, abnormal venous blood flow and vascular damage.

18.1.2.1 Altered coagulation

Factor VIII and von Willibrand factors increase three to four times in pregnancy promoting coagulation. Protein S, an anticoagulant, decreases in the mid first trimester and remains low until a few weeks postpartum. Fibrinolysis is reduced due to the increase in the plasminogen activator inhibitor. These clotting changes are all pro-coagulant.

18.1.2.2 Abnormal venous flow

As the gravid uterus increases in size, venous return progressively decreases, leading to venous pooling and stasis in the iliac and lower limb vessels. In addition, the pregnancy hormone oestrogen causes vascular smooth muscle distension and further venous pooling.

18.1.2.3 Vascular damage

Endothelial damage occurs at the point of the right iliac artery crossing the left iliac vein. Oestrogen mediated venous distension leads to endothelial disruption. Endothelial damage to the pelvic veins occurs at the time of delivery, which explains the increased risk of VTE postpartum.

18.1.3 Diagnosis of deep vein thrombosis (DVT)

An accurate diagnosis of DVT is very important in pregnancy to prevent the unnecessary exposure of the mother and the fetus to anticoagulant therapy, which may have consequences for management of delivery, and prevent progression to a catastrophic pulmonary embolism.

18.1.3.1 Clinical features

Typical features include leg pain, skin discolouration in the legs, unilateral leg swelling.

18.1.3.2 Investigations

Clinical suspicion of a DVT should ideally be followed by further investigations as available: D-dimer blood test, direct ultrasound imaging for echogenic thrombus, doppler flow of pelvic veins, venography without an abdominal shield (safe fetal radiation exposure) or CT venography (high fetal radiation exposure).

The usefulness of D-dimer in pregnancy is limited by the normal physiologic increase in pregnancy, which causes a high proportion of false positive results.

18.1.4 Diagnosis of pulmonary embolus (PE)

The diagnosis of pulmonary embolism can be made from typical clinical features, a ventilation perfusion (VQ) lung scan or computed tomographic pulmonary angiography (CTPA) depending on available resources.

18.1.4.1 Clinical features

The common symptoms of PE are sudden onset of cough, dyspnoea, pleuritic chest pain, and haemoptysis. Central chest pain, hypotension, convulsions, and cardiac arrest can occur in massive PE. Sinus tachycardia and crepitations on chest auscultation may be the only clinical findings. A pleural rub may be apparent on examination. Following a massive PE, evidence of right ventricular failure with jugular venous distension, liver enlargement, and a parasternal heave can occur.

18.1.4.2 Investigations

Due to the lack of sophisticated X-Ray facilities and also concerns regarding fetal exposure to radiation, simple methods have been suggested for initial management. In a mother with a strong clinical suspicion of PE, direct ultrasound imaging of the iliac and leg veins should be the first test considered. A positive test will infer PE and any further radiation exposure can be avoided.

If ultrasound of the legs and pelvic veins is negative, a VQ scan should be performed. A normal VQ scan excludes a PE, however 50–60% of VQ scans are not conclusive and further investigation is required.

18.1.5 Management of VTE

Anticoagulant therapy is the mainstay of treatment; however, there are significant safety concerns for the mother and fetus. Low molecular weight heparin (LMWH) and unfractionated heparin (UFH) are both safe for the fetus during pregnancy, but treatment can cause maternal bleeding, osteoporosis, heparin induced thrombocytopaenia and allergic skin reactions. Warfarin therapy can lead to fetal abnormalities and intra-uterine death.

18.1.5.1 Treatment of acute VTE

- LMWH once or twice a day by subcutaneous injection
- UFH every 12 hours by subcutaneous injection to obtain a therapeutic range activated partial thromboplastin time (APTT) i.e. APTT ratio of 1.5–2.5
- In extensive disease with a potentially unstable mother, an intravenous infusion of UFH following a bolus dose, with a target APTT ratio of 1.5–2.5.

18.1.5.2 Labour and delivery

Any mother receiving anticoagulant therapy during pregnancy will be at high risk of haemorrhage at the time of delivery, unless her anticoagulant treatment is reduced or stopped in the hours before delivery. The residual effects of UFH and LMWH can be seen for at least 24 hours after the last therapeutic dose. Therefore, labour and delivery should be planned in advance. If there are any doubts regarding the coagulation status, regional anaesthetic techniques should not be performed due to the increased risk of spinal or epidural haematoma.

Following delivery, LMWH or UFH should be recommenced 12–24 hours after delivery if there are no bleeding concerns.

Warfarin should be initiated after adequate haemostasis with bridging UFH or LMWH therapy to achieve the target international normalized ratio (INR) of 2 and continued for between 6–12 weeks post-delivery.

18.1.6 Venous thrombo-embolism prophylaxis

During the postpartum period, mothers are at high risk of developing VTE due to their pro-coagulant state and reduced mobility. The following should be used as a guide for prophylaxis of VTE.

Table 18.1 Venous thrombo-embolism prophylaxis

	Enoxaparin (100units/mg)	Dalteparin	Tinzaparin
Normal body weight	40mg daily	5000 units daily	4500 units daily
Body weight < 50 kg	20mg daily	2500 units daily	3500 units daily
Body weight > 90 kg	40mg 12 hourly	5000 units 12 hourly	4500 units 12 hourly

18.2 Amniotic fluid embolism (AFE)

AFE is a rare but devastating condition, where amniotic fluid enters the pulmonary circulation causing rapid and profound effects on gas exchange and frequently leading to maternal cardio-respiratory arrest. Coagulopathy occurs within minutes and has a reported mortality of greater than 50%. The risk factors for AFE include multi-parity, trauma in late pregnancy, a precipitous labour or delivery of a large baby, placental abruption, or caesarean section delivery.

18.2.1 Clinical features

Typical clinical features include acute dyspnoea, sudden development of a mottled rash, cardiovascular collapse and severe clotting abnormality.

18.2.2 Diagnosis

The diagnosis of AFE is usually made after all other causes of cardio-vascular collapse have been excluded. The differential diagnosis includes: PE, haemorrhage, massive air embolism, anaphylaxis and acute myocardial infarction. However, there should be a high index of suspicion if the mother becomes hypoxic, hypotensive and develops a sudden and severe coagulopathy.

18.2.3 Management

Supportive therapy is the mainstay of treatment following an ABC approach. Any ongoing haemorrhage should be promptly treated with intravenous fluids and blood, and clotting abnormalities corrected.

18.3 Air embolism

Massive air embolism is rare but potentially lethal. Air is entrained into the circulation via the open venous plexus of the placental bed at the time of placental separation. Minor air emboli are probably very common and account for the sensation of chest tightness or heaviness frequently seen immediately following delivery in awake patients. However, air may also enter the circulation via IV lines, which have not been primed with IV fluid correctly. Symptoms may be evident when greater than 0.5 ml/kg/min of air has entered the circulation.

18.3.1 Clinical features

The clinical features are similar to an AFE without deranged coagulation. If the patient has an undiagnosed patent foramen ovale, additional features would include neurological manifestations, i.e. hemiparesis and seizures, as the air emboli crosses into the systemic circulation.

18.3.2 **Management**

The surgical area should be flooded with saline if an air embolism is suspected at CS. All IV lines should be re-checked for the presence of air. The mainstay of management is supportive, with an ABC approach. An IV fluid bolus and vasopressors should be given to increase the central venous pressure and force the air out of the pulmonary circulation.

Chapter 19

Anaesthesia and analgesia for specific obstetric conditions

Sarah Harries

Key points

- The obstetric anaesthetist is requested to deal with a variety of problems on a busy delivery suite each day
- An understanding of the common obstetric problems is essential to safely provide the appropriate anaesthetic management
- Teamwork and prompt, effective communication between anaesthetists, anaesthetic practitioners, midwives, and obstetricians are vital in each situation
- It is important for all professionals involved to understand their own role and the factors affecting the decision-making of other disciplines.

19.1 Intra-uterine death

The unexpected death of a fetus after 20 weeks gestation may be detected by a prolonged period of absent fetal movements and confirmed by the absence of a fetal heart-beat on Doppler or preferably ultrasound scanning. The underlying maternal or fetal cause is frequently not found.

19.1.1 Key issues

Intra-uterine death is a devastating event for parents and the management of the subsequent delivery is emotionally difficult and stressful for all staff involved. There are major obstetric consequences: deranged clotting, sepsis, postpartum haemorrhage.

Labour is usually induced as soon as feasible after the diagnosis has been confirmed, with the aim to deliver the fetus vaginally. Labour may be prolonged and difficult, especially if the fetus is near term gestation and may require assisted delivery.

19.1.2 **Management**

The mother should be assessed for signs of a coagulopathy or sepsis prior to discussion of pain relief available for delivery. You should record: serial temperature, pulse rate and blood pressure, and check FBC and clotting. Any clotting abnormalities should be corrected. Any signs of infection should be treated with broad spectrum antibiotics, e.g. IV penicillins and metronidazole. Regional techniques are contra-indicated if a coagulopathy is present or uncorrected.

19.2 **Breech presentation**

The position of the fetus at term is defined by its lie i.e. the relationship of the longitudinal axis of the fetus to that of the mother, and the nature of the presenting part foremost in the pelvis, e.g. cephalic (head), breech (buttock), compound or abnormal lie.

19.2.1 Key issues

Breech presentation and abnormal lie are both associated with grand multiparity, polyhydramnios, placenta previa, and other obstructive lesions in the pelvis, e.g. large uterine fibroids. There is an increased risk of cord prolapse and consequently fetal compromise. If a mother presents with a mal-presentation, early anaesthetic assessment of the mother is important because of the high incidence of intervention often required. Effective teamwork between obstetrician, anaesthetist, and midwife is essential to ensure a safe delivery and best outcome for mother and baby.

19.2.2 Management of breech presentation

Vaginal breech delivery has been shown to be associated with greater intrapartum hypoxia than a vaginal, cephalic delivery, due to prolonged compression of the umbilical cord during the second stage of labour. If a breech presentation persists until term, it is now recognized that perinatal mortality, neonatal mortality and serious neonatal morbidity are significantly lower following a planned caesarean section (CS) compared to a planned vaginal breech delivery. As a result, many women opt for an external cephalic version (ECV), where the aim is to turn the fetus around to a cephalic position before labour starts, or a planned CS if an ECV fails.

19.2.2.1 Labour management

Continuous fetal monitoring is essential throughout labour, with the facilities available to proceed to emergency CS if required. The anaesthetist should remain near to the delivery room to deal swiftly with any complications.

19.2.2.2 Caesarean section

There are many situations when a CS may be required for breech presentation: planned CS, emergency CS following a known or undiagnosed breech presenting in labour or if there is severe fetal distress during a planned vaginal breech delivery. Regional anaesthesia confers significant benefits over GA for CS and should be attempted if time allows. If an emergency CS is required during the second stage of labour, extraction of the fetus may be very difficult at CS. Additional uterine relaxation may be required, e.g. 50–100mcg IV glyceryl (GTN) or sublingual GTN spray.

19.3 Vaginal delivery after CS (VBAC)

If a woman has undergone a transverse incision caesarean section for a previous delivery, subsequent vaginal delivery is possible (VBAC).

19.3.1 Key issues

VBAC is safe and effective in carefully selected mothers and has a success rate of 72–76%. Repeat elective CS is also safe, but does carry additional risks e.g. haemorrhage, thromboembolism, bladder damage and adhesions. Contraindications to VBAC include: previous classical incision CS, extensive uterine surgery, previous uterine rupture, 3 or more CS. The main risk is uterine dehiscence or rupture during labour. Extreme caution is advised with the use of induction agents, e.g. prostaglandins and oxytocics.

19.3.2 Complications

The main complication is uterine scar rupture, which can present with: severe abdominal pain which is continuous in nature, intra-partum bleeding, maternal tachycardia, hypotension or collapse, fetal distress, or demise. Management includes immediate delivery by CS and prompt resuscitation of the mother.

19.4 Fetal distress

The most important thing to appreciate when dealing with cases of 'fetal distress' is that this term covers a wide range of degrees of risk to the fetus. The diagnosis of intra-partum fetal distress usually indicates that the obstetrician considers the fetus needs early or immediate delivery and the timing of delivery is graded according to the following categories for CS:

- Category 1: 'Decision to delivery' time 15–30 minutes
- Category 2: 'Decision to delivery' time less than 1 hour
- Category 3: 'Decision to delivery' time less than 24 hours
- Category 4: 'Decision to delivery' time to suit staff.

19.4.1 **Key issues**

Effective teamwork and communication is essential. Discuss the patient with the obstetrician, midwives and obstetric theatre team.

Ascertain the degree of urgency immediately. The mother is your first priority and as her anaesthetist, her safety is your prime concern. In difficult situations, everyone else will be focused on the baby and you may be the sole voice for the mother. Don't be afraid to speak up for her.

During transfer to theatre, every effort should be made to improve the fetal condition and provide 'intra-uterine resuscitation', which includes: position the mother in full left lateral to reduce aorto-caval compression, administer oxygen by face mask, treat hypotension with increments of vasopressor, e.g. IV ephedrine or adrenaline, stop oxytocic drug infusions, consider tocolytic drugs, e.g. IV terbutaline 100–250mcg, IV GTN 50mcg or sublingual GTN 200–400mcg. Always reassess the situation with the obstetrician after transfer to theatre. Reapply the CTG monitor—if fetal heart is more reassuring, the options for the anaesthetic technique for delivery should be discussed again.

19.4.2 **Management of delivery**

The management of 'fetal distress' depends on the stage of labour and the degree of concern. It is essential to establish immediately with the obstetrician the required 'decision to delivery' time.

19.4.2.1 *First stage of labour*

'Fetal distress' during first stage almost always necessitates delivery by emergency CS. General anesthesia is usually required for a Category 1 section when the mother's life is in danger or the 'decision to delivery' time is less than 15 minutes. An experienced anaesthetist may decide to have ONE attempt inserting a spinal anaesthetic, whilst the woman is being pre-oxygenated via a tight-fitting mask and the fetus monitored continuously. If the attempt is successful, the caesarean section may proceed; however, there must be a low threshold for stopping and no time lost before converting to a GA. The degree of urgency following the decision for CS can change in either direction, therefore it is vital that the fetal heart is monitored closely.

19.4.2.2 *Second stage of labour*

Fetal distress in the second stage occurs not infrequently when the vertex is visible. This is often successfully managed with experienced midwifery care. If fetal distress occurs in the second stage of labour, when the fetus is below the ischial spines, an emergency assisted ventouse or outlet forceps delivery in the delivery room may be appropriate. This can be performed under a pudendal nerve block: 10 mls of 1% lidocaine is injected just below and medial to the ischial spines bilaterally and it should be supplemented with perineal infiltration for the episiotomy. If the obstetrician considers a 'trial of instrumental delivery' to be appropriate, the woman should be transferred rapidly to theatre with fetal monitoring in place. If the decision to delivery time is less than 15 minutes, the most appropriate decision is an emergency CS. It is essential that the degree of urgency for CS is discussed before deciding on a particular anaesthetic technique.

19.4.3 **Recognition of the 'at risk' fetus**

Regular communication with the midwives and obstetricians is of paramount importance to enable you to spot the 'At Risk' fetus and form an early management plan of 'what to do if...' in your mind. Attend staff handover rounds and have regular updates on new admissions. Watch out for: slow labour, induced or augmented with syntocinon, pre-eclampsia, intrauterine growth retardation ('small for dates'), meconium staining of liquor.

19.5 **Placental abruption**

Placental abruption is premature separation of a normally implanted placenta.

19.5.1 **Key issues**

There are many associated risk factors: pre-eclampsia, eclampsia or chronic hypertension, premature rupture of membranes, increased uterine size, e.g. multiple pregnancy, polyhydramnios, multi-parity. Classical signs include: abdominal pain, haemorrhage, uterine tenderness or irritability, coagulopathy or fetal distress, or demise. The presence of abdominal pain often differentiates an abruption from bleeding secondary to a placenta previa. It may present with either profound revealed or concealed bleeding, requiring rapid resuscitation of the mother. Blood loss with a concealed retro-placental haemtoma is frequently under-estimated. Close observation of the mother is required as cardiovascular stability is often maintained until >40% of the circulating blood volume is lost (2–3 L).

Clotting abnormalities occur early following an abruption. Prompt correction of a coagulopathy is necessary to minimize further bleeding. Stabilization of the mother and immediate delivery can be life-saving for the mother and fetus. The perinatal mortality rate following a major placental abruption can be as high as 50%.

19.5.2 **Management**

Establish IV access with 2 large bore cannulae and commence fluid resuscitation, administer oxygen by face mask and send blood for urgent FBC, clotting studies and cross-match 2–4 units of blood, depending on the degree of concern. Rapid assessment of the cardiovascular status of the mother, and viability and gestational age of the fetus is important, as this will determine the ultimate obstetric management of delivery.

19.5.2.1 Viable fetus

If bleeding is continuing and/or the fetus demonstrates signs of distress, immediate delivery by CS is indicated. CS should not be delayed until blood results, cross-matched blood or blood products are available if the mother or fetus remains compromised in any way.

General anaesthesia is the technique of choice for the mother who is cardiovascularly compromised, or a coagulopathy is present. Regional anaesthesia is not contra-indicated provided the mother is not hypovolaemic and there is no evidence of clotting abnormalities. A single-shot spinal technique would be appropriate. Despite the urgency, it is important to complete a rapid pre-operative anaesthetic assessment and not forget to administer antacid prophylaxis.

19.5.2.2 Dead fetus

If the placental separation has caused intra-uterine death, vaginal delivery is the preferred mode of delivery, provided there is no ongoing catastrophic maternal haemorrhage. Following resuscitation, any coagulopathy should be corrected.

19.5.2.3 Postoperative complications

Always exclude co-existing pre-eclampsia when faced with a placental abruption. The fluid management can be difficult to manage effectively and the mother can rapidly develop pulmonary oedema. The risk of uterine atony following delivery is increased. At CS, all blood clots should be fully evacuated from the uterus and the uterus massaged to aid contraction. Additional uterotonics may be required to maintain uterine contraction, e.g. IV/IM ergometrine, IV oxytocin infusion or misoprostol PR. Disseminated intravascular coagulation (DIC) complicates ~10% of all abruptions but is more common if fetal death has occurred. Acute renal failure may result if DIC or hypovolaemia remains uncorrected.

19.6 Cord prolapse

Cord prolapse occurs when the umbilical cord lies in front of or beside the presenting part, in the presence of ruptured membranes.

19.6.1 Key issues

Cord prolapse is an obstetric emergency, as compression of the umbilical cord will severely compromise the fetal bood supply and precipitate immediate fetal distress. Delivery by CS must be performed extremely quickly, i.e. within minutes, to ensure no hypoxic damage to the fetus. Predisposing factors include: high/ill fitting presenting part, breech, high parity, prematurity, multiple pregnancy, polyhydramnios, high head at the time of either spontaneous or instrumental membrane rupture.

19.6.2 Management

Although speed is essential, the situation should not prevent a rapid pre-operative assessment prior to CS and antacid prophylaxis. Oxygen must be administered via a tight fitting face mask. For transfer to theatre, the presenting part must be pushed out of the pelvis with manual upward pressure by the obstetrician or midwife. If fetal blood supply remains compromised, general anaesthesia is the only option and a standard technique is applied with the usual safety precautions. The drugs required for a GA should always be prepared in advance and refrigerated, ready for a Category 1 CS. Simulated drills of cord prolapse involving the delivery suite and theatre team should be performed regularly and any weak points from the drills addressed.

19.7 Twins and other multiple pregnancies

The incidence of twin pregnancies is 1 in 80, triplets 1 in 8000 and quads 1 in 800,000.

19.7.1 Key issues

Multiple pregnancies are associated with a number of major obstetric complications, placing them at increased risk during pregnancy and delivery: pre-eclampsia, anaemia, intrauterine death, malpresentations, premature labour, prolonged labour, malpresentation of second twin following delivery of first twin, postpartum haemorrhage secondary to uterine atony. Aorto-caval compression is much more severe.

19.7.2 Management

In a twin pregnancy, if the first twin is cephalic presentation and there is no evidence of other co-existing problems, there is often no reason why these women cannot labour. In triplet and quadruplet pregnancies, a planned CS between 34–36 weeks gestation is the preferred mode of delivery, before preterm labour is threatened.

19.7.2.1 Labour

The labour may be long, and the second fetus may present abnormally, necessitating instrumental delivery, cephalic version, or immediate CS. The anaesthetist should be aware at all times of the progress of labour in twin births, and be present during the second stage of labour to respond and treat appropriately if the decision is made to transfer to theatre or for emergency CS.

19.7.2.2 Caesarean section

The usual choices for anaesthetic technique apply. The subarachnoid space may be compressed increasing the risk of a high spinal block, therefore the dose of intrathecal local anaesthetic should be reduced by 20%. Aorto-caval compression is greater and hypotension following a spinal block is likely to be more severe, therefore maintain left lateral position for as long as possible following insertion of the regional technique. Large-bore venous access, close observation and additional oxytocics are recommended to treat uterine atony.

19.8 Premature fetus

The premature fetus is defined as a delivery between 20 and 37 weeks gestation.

19.8.1 Key issues

Risk factors for pre-term delivery include: previous pre-term delivery, multiple pregnancy, infection (e.g. chorio-amnionitis, pyelonephritis), abnormal placentation (e.g placenta previa, extremes of age). To improve fetal lung maturity, two doses of steroid, e.g. beta-methasone, 12 hours apart, are beneficial if administered to the mother when the gestational age is less than 34 weeks. If possible, delivery should be delayed until 24 hours after the first dose.

19.8.2 Management

Labour may progress rapidly but if a CS is required, a 'Classical' CS with a vertical incision in the uterus may be necessary if the gestational age is less than 28 weeks, as the lower segment of the uterus has not developed at this stage. A regional anaesthetic technique is appropriate for either a Classical or lower segment CS; however, the dose of local anaesthetic required to provide an adequate block will be greater than that required for a term CS by about 20%. In the extreme pre-term situation, syntocinon may not be fully effective in promoting uterine contraction as the receptors are not fully developed. Ergometrine is more suitable post delivery to prevent uterine atony.

19.9 Placenta praevia

Placenta praevia occurs when the placenta either completely or partially covers the internal cervical os, or is implanted at its margin. It is associated with considerable morbidity and mortality. The incidence is approximately 1 in 200 pregnancies, but is higher with previous uterine scars, multiparity and increasing maternal age.

19.9.1 **Key issues**

Placenta previa can present with painless insidious vaginal bleeding, catastrophic obstetric haemorrhage or be asymptomatic. The differential diagnosis is placental abruption, which is usually associated with abdominal pain and uterine tenderness or irritability. An ultrasound will differentiate these two diagnoses.

Postpartum haemorrhage is a major risk. Early use of ergometrine, continuous syntocinon infusion, misoprostol PR, and carboprost should be considered. If bleeding is uncontrolled following delivery, early use of a B-Lynch suture +/- an intra-uterine balloon device may avoid the need for a caesarean hysterectomy.

19.9.2 **Management**

19.9.2.1 Initial resuscitation

Following presentation with a vaginal bleed, an urgent ultrasound will confirm the diagnosis and the position of the previa. In the event of major haemorrhage, two large bore cannulae should be inserted and fluid resuscitation commenced. Blood should be sent for FBC, clotting studies and cross-matched blood requested.

19.9.2.2 Elective CS

Whenever possible, elective caesarean section is delayed until 38 weeks to reduce neonatal morbidity. Traditionally, regional anaesthesia has been relatively contra-indicated for an elective CS for major previas, particularly anterior placenta previas, and general anaesthesia advocated because of the risk of uncontrolled bleeding. A senior anaesthetist and obstetrician should be present for the CS. Two large bore cannulae should be inserted prior to starting surgery and invasive BP monitoring is recommended for a major anterior previa. Major haemorrhage during surgery should be anticipated. Cross-matched blood should be available in theatre or in the delivery suite fridge prior to surgery. Resuscitation of the mother will be optimized by the use of rapid infusion devices, with the facility to warm all infusion fluids.

19.2.2.3 Emergency CS

General anaesthesia should be performed in any mother with uncontrolled bleeding despite resuscitation, any cardiovascular instability, coagulopathy, or fetal distress. Ideally, an experienced anaesthetist and obstetrician should take responsibility for the surgery.

Resuscitation should continue throughout transfer to theatre and preparation for general anaesthesia. It is not advisable to start surgery before blood is available for rapid infusion at the time of uterine incision.

19.10 **Suturing the perineum**

Perineal trauma may occur spontaneously during vaginal birth or by surgical incision, i.e. episiotomy, where an incision is intentionally made to increase the diameter of the vulval outlet to facilitate delivery. 1st and 2nd degree tears involve the skin and perineal muscles, 3rd and 4th degree tears involve the anal sphincter and epithelium and require expert repair.

19.10.1 **Key issues**

There are a number of recognized risk factors for perineal trauma: fetal birth weight >4000g, prolonged 2nd stage of labour, instrumental delivery, direct occipito-posterior position, nutritional status. Perineal trauma can be associated with significant post-delivery haemorrhage, which is often under-estimated. Continuing vaginal bleeding should always be investigated. High vaginal or cervical lacerations may be missed and continued bleeding falsely attributed to uterine atony. Perineal trauma causes significant pain and discomfort in the early post-delivery period and in the longer term, with urinary and faecal incontinence. Examination and suturing should be performed as soon as possible to reduce bleeding, pain and the risk of infection.

19.10.2 **Management**

Assess the mother for signs of hypovolaemia, establish IV access, check FBC +/− clotting studies, and request cross-matched blood early. Superficial suturing of the perineum is usually performed with local infiltration instilled by the obstetrician or midwife. More extensive suturing of the perineum usually requires transfer to the operating theatre for further assessment and both anaesthetic and surgical management.

A low spinal is required (e.g. 1.5–2 ml heavy 0.5% bupivacaine +/− short-acting opioid). Site the spinal with the mother in the lateral position if she is uncomfortable, and sit her up or with 45° head up tilt as soon as possible thereafter. General anaesthesia may be necessary to achieve adequate muscle relaxation and visualisation for surgical repair of severe or complex lacerations, or for delayed or revision of suturing. General anaesthesia is also best for the haemodynamically unstable mother or if a coagulopathy prevents a regional technique. Antacid prophylaxis should be given and a rapid sequence induction performed on all mothers requiring general anaesthesia within 24 hours of delivery. Beware of opioid analgesia causing constipation and straining at defaecation. A regular laxative should be prescribed with all opioids.

19.11 **Retained placenta**

The third stage of labour involves the separation, descent and delivery of the placenta. The placenta is considered retained if it fails to deliver within 60 minutes of birth.

19.11.1 **Key issues**

Retained placenta is a common cause of postpartum haemorrhage, with an incidence of ~2%. It is a significant cause of maternal morbidity and mortality world-wide. Potential complications include: primary and secondary (delayed) postpartum haemorrhage, 'cervical shock' (i.e. profound bradycardia and hypotension precipitated by increased vagal tone when the placenta sits in the open cervix) and uterine inversion.

19.11.2 **Management**

19.11.2.1 *Early management*

Initial management may be conservative. Empty the bladder and wait for signs of spontaneous separation and delivery of the placenta.

Early initiation of breast-feeding may assist placental separation. Active management of 3rd stage involves use of available uterotonics with controlled cord traction after uterine contraction. A second dose of uterotonic may be required. Blood loss may be concealed and close observation for maternal pallor, tachycardia and hypotension must be maintained. Establish IV access with a large bore cannula, estimate amount and rate of blood loss and cardiovascular stability, and check FBC +/− clotting studies and arrange for cross-matched blood. If the placenta has not been expelled after an hour or there is significant bleeding +/− haemodynamic instability, the placenta must be removed manually.

19.11.2.2 *Manual removal of placenta*

Manual removal of placenta should be performed in the theatre environment, preferably under regional anaesthesia, provided no contra-indications exist, e.g. uncorrected hypovolaemia or coagulopathy. A sensory block to T6 is required for pain-free manual removal of placenta as the uterine fundus is often manipulated (e.g. 2.5 ml heavy 0.5% bupivacaine +/− short-acting opioid). Site the spinal with the mother in the lateral position if she is uncomfortable. Continuous monitoring of ECG and pulse oximetry, and intermittent BP should always be performed.

General anaesthesia may be required for the haemodynamically unstable mother or if a coagulopathy prevents a regional technique. Antacid prophylaxis should be given and a standard rapid sequence induction performed. A volatile agent will assist placenta removal by providing greater uterine relaxation but may also increase bleeding.

On placental delivery, administer available uterotonics, e.g. 5 IU oxytocin IV bolus (caution if patient is hypotensive) followed by an infusion of 40 IU oxytocin in 500 ml normal saline over 4 hours.

19.12 **Uterine inversion**

Puerperal uterine inversion is the displacement of the fundus of the uterus usually occurring during the 3rd stage of labour. Although rare, it is a serious, life-threatening emergency due to associated blood loss and cardiovascular instability.

19.12.1 **Key issues**

The classical presentation of uterine inversion is an obviously displaced uterus during placental delivery, postpartum haemorrhage, severe pain and clinical shock, which appears out of proportion to the blood loss. Shock is thought to be due, in part, to the parasympathetic response to traction on the uterine suspensory ligaments and often accompanied by profound bradycardia. This is an emergency and there should be no delay in instituting treatment.

19.12.2 **Management**

Simultaneously treat haemorrhagic shock (i.e. high flow oxygen, aggressive IV fluid resuscitation), give atropine for bradycardia, and replace the uterus. Any delay in replacement will increase uterine oedema, impeding later replacement and exacerbate cardiovascular instability. Immediate general anaesthesia is usually required to facilitate uterine replacement. The uterus may be replaced manually or by hydrostatic correction, pouring warm saline into the vagina. Tocolytic drugs can be given to increase cervical relaxation:

- β2 receptor agonists—Salbutamol 0.25mg i.v. bolus
- Magnesium sulphate—4 g i.v. over 10 minutes.
- Glyceryl trinitrate—50–100mcg i.v. bolus.

Volatile general anaesthetic agents will cause uterine and cervical relaxation. Severe cases may require laparotomy and combined abdominal-vaginal correction.

Chapter 20

Intrauterine fetal resuscitation and newborn resuscitation

Isabeau Walker, Zipporah Gathuya

Key points

- Many situations where newborn babies require resuscitation can be predicted
- Intrauterine fetal resuscitation may buy additional time to plan an emergency delivery where fetal distress is present
- The key interventions in intrauterine fetal resuscitation are to place the mother in the left lateral position and to administer high flow oxygen
- All babies need to be dried, gently stimulated and assessed immediately after birth
- The key intervention in newborn resuscitation is effective ventilation of the lungs
- Anyone who delivers a baby should be capable of basic newborn resuscitation.

20.1 Introduction

The majority of newborn babies require minimal intervention at birth to establish normal breathing and transition to extra-uterine life. However, on a global scale, many babies still die during labour (intrapartum-related stillbirth), or early in the neonatal period (intrapartum-related neonatal death). It is estimated that there are 2 million perinatal deaths every year, with 99% occurring in low-and middle-income countries. There are an estimated one million survivors of birth asphyxia who go on to develop cerebral palsy, learning difficulties or who have other disabilities.

Many cases of death and disability in newborns can be prevented by:
- Early recognition of the at-risk pregnancy
- Timely intervention for the complicated labour, including intrauterine fetal resuscitation.
- Immediate resuscitation of the 'at risk' baby and those who do not breathe effectively at birth.

This chapter will consider interventions to improve outcomes for newborn infants in resource-limited settings.

20.2 **Recognition of the at risk pregnancy**

Obstructed labour and malpresentation represent the commonest risk to the newborn, particularly when associated with delay in diagnosis or accessing care. A number of factors predict the need for newborn resuscitation on a population basis.

Maternal factors include:
- Maternal age <18 years, >35 years
- Maternal size <150cm or pre-pregnancy weight <47 kg
- Primigravida or parity >6
- Poor obstetric history (previous perinatal death or instrumental delivery).

Factors arising during pregnancy include:
- Multiple pregnancy
- Maternal anaemia
- Maternal jaundice
- Pre-eclampsia and eclampsia
- Diabetes
- Syphilis
- Maternal malaria (blood test positive)
- HIV especially when combined with malaria
- Post-term (>42 weeks) and preterm birth (<37 weeks gestation)
- Maternal drug abuse.

Factors arising during labour and childbirth:
- Obstructed labour and prolonged second stage
- Meconium staining of liquor
- Prolapsed cord
- Breech presentation or other malpresentations
- PV bleeding after the 8th month
- Maternal fever during labour (>38°C)
- Rupture membranes > 24 hours
- Poor maternal effort and need for instrumental delivery.

20.3 **Monitoring during labour**

All women in labour should be routinely monitored to assess progress and the response of the fetus to labour, in particular to detect fetal distress due to fetal hypoxia. The fetal heart rate should be monitored at baseline and in response to uterine contractions. Low-risk patients should be monitored hourly during active labour; high risk patients should be monitored half-hourly or more frequently if fetal distress is detected.

A number of methods of monitoring during labour are in use in resource-poor settings:

- Partogram—Paper form to record regular assessments of maternal and fetal condition during active labour. Useful to identify when values vary from the normal range
- Fetal kick chart—Mother keeps a record of fetal movement
- Pinard stethoscope—Handheld stethoscope used for intermittent assessment of the fetal heart rate
- Umbilical artery Doppler—Detects umbilical artery waveforms by Doppler ultrasound. Abnormal waveforms indicate poor placental perfusion and may be used to assess fetal well-being in early labour
- Cardiotocography (CTG)—Doppler ultrasound to detect the fetal heart rate and a strain gauge to assess uterine contractions. Gives continuous assessment of the fetus and labour in high-risk patients, but requires training to interpret. It is complex equipment, which is expensive to purchase and maintain
- Fetal blood sampling—Blood samples taken from the fetal scalp. Useful only after rupture of membranes and carries a risk of infection to the fetus in areas of high prevalence of HIV/hepatitis. It is the 'Gold-standard' to assess fetal wellbeing, but expensive and rarely available
- Assessment of liquor—Meconium staining of liquor indicates that either fetal distress is present or that there is risk of fetal distress. The fetal heart rate should be assessed to plan appropriate action. The infant is likely to require active resuscitation at birth.

Estimation of the fetal heart rate is an essential component of the assessment of fetal wellbeing. If the fetus becomes hypoxic during labour, this will result in fetal distress and bradycardia. A baseline bradycardia or late decelerations are particularly concerning and are an indication for fetal resuscitation and expedited delivery. Normal fetal heart rate is 110–150 beats/min, with normal beat-to-beat variation of at least 5 beats/min.

- A baseline tachycardia is moderate if >150 and severe if >170 beats/min. This may be due to maternal pyrexia, exhaustion, chorioamnionitis, fetal distress, fetal haemorrhage, or anaemia

- Baseline bradycardia (<100 beats/min)—This indicates severe fetal distress due to fetal hypoxia. If there are also decelerations, there is a high risk of fetal death.
- Loss of baseline variability with a flat trace on the cardiotocograph. This indicates possible fetal distress or possibly the fetus is sleeping or effect of maternal analgesics—monitor carefully
- Early decelerations where the fetal heart rate decreases during a contraction, but returns to normal by the end of the contraction is a natural vagal response caused by compression of the fetal head during a contraction. It indicates an increased risk of fetal distress—monitor closely
- Late deceleration where the fetal heart rate decreases during a contraction with delayed return to baseline (>30 seconds after contraction has ended). This pattern indicates fetal distress due to hypoxia
- Variable deceleration is a deceleration unrelated to contractions. It is usually caused by compression of the umbilical cord—monitor closely.

20.4 **Intrauterine fetal resuscitation**

Intrauterine fetal resuscitation is essential in all situations where there is fetal distress with baseline fetal bradycardia with or without late decelerations. Catastrophic fetal compromise requiring immediate resuscitation may be seen in placental abruption or placenta previa, uterine rupture, umbilical cord prolapse or fetal haemorrhage from vasa previa (umbilical vessels passing in front of the cervical os).

Intrauterine fetal resuscitation improves oxygen delivery to the fetus by increasing the oxygen content of placental blood, and by restoring blood flow to the fetus through the umbilical vessels.

Immediate steps:

- Place the mother in full left or right lateral position to avoid maternal supine hypotension. The mother should kneel forwards on her elbows if cord prolapse is suspected as this takes the pressure of the presenting part off the umbilical cord
- Administer high flow oxygen to the mother using a well-fitting oxygen mask with reservoir bag.

Consider:

- 1000 ml Ringers/Hartmann's or Normal Saline IV to increase maternal blood pressure (caution in pre-eclampsia)
- Vasoconstrictor (e.g. ephedrine 6mg IV) if maternal hypotension is due to extensive sympathetic block from regional anaesthesia.
- Stop oxytocic agents to reduce uterine activity (if in use)
- Tocolytic agent (e.g. terbutaline 250mcg SC or GTN sublingual spray, 2 puffs initially, repeat after 1 minute, maximum 3 doses).

The obstetric team should make simultaneous preparations for immediate delivery (less than 30 minutes), either by vaginal delivery or by caesarean section. Intrauterine resuscitation may restore the fetal heart rate and buy additional time to plan the delivery, and may also improve fetal outcomes. Active resuscitation of the newborn should be expected.

20.5 Newborn resuscitation

All babies require immediate assessment at birth and to be dried and covered and kept warm, preferably by skin-to-skin contact with the mother. In the vast majority of cases, these simple interventions suffice. Around 10% of babies require assistance to start breathing and 1% require more extensive resuscitation – this figure may be higher in areas where prolonged labour or late presentation are common.

Situations where babies commonly require active resuscitation include:

- Fetal distress during labour
- Prematurity
- Abnormal presentation
- Difficult or traumatic delivery
- General anaesthesia or recent opioid analgesia
- Maternal drug abuse, especially alcohol
- Babies of diabetic mothers
- Small for gestational age babies
- Prolonged rupture of membranes where infection is suspected.

However, it is not always possible to predict which babies will require assistance, so it is essential that anyone who delivers a baby should be able to perform resuscitation and that the facilities for newborn resuscitation are available at every delivery.

Newborn resuscitation is usually the responsibility of the midwives, although in some units there may be dedicated paediatricians available for complex cases. The prime responsibility of the anaesthetist during a caesarean section is the care of the mother, but the knowledge and skills of the anaesthetist may be invaluable in resuscitation of the newborn. The anaesthetist should therefore train with the midwives on a regular basis to develop their resuscitation skills.

20.5.1 Preparation of the environment for delivery

The baby should be delivered in a clean environment away from drafts. There should be clean instruments to cut and tie the cord. The room temperature should be maintained at 25°C or there should be a source of heat. There should be a good light source to assess the baby, and hand washing facilities to reduce infection.

20.5.2 **Preparation for resuscitation of the newborn**

The equipment listed below should be routinely available and checked every day.

Essential equipment includes: a source of heat e.g. heater, lamp or resuscitaire; warm, dry linen; scissors, strapping, tapes; self-inflating bag (500ml infant size); anaesthetic face masks–sizes 0 and 1.

Equipment recommended as desirable includes: stethoscope; suction equipment (Yankauer suction and suction catheters size 6, 7, and 8); oxygen source, flow meter, oxygen tubing; syringes and needles/swabs.

More specialist equipment includes: Oral airways size 000, 00 and 0; neonatal laryngoscope with spare batteries and bulb; tracheal tubes size 2.5, 3.0 and 3.5; umbilical catheters (or sterile size 4 nasogastric tube); 1:10,000 adrenaline; 4.2% sodium bicarbonate; 10% dextrose.

20.5.3 **Physiological principles of newborn resuscitation**

It is normal for the fetus to experience transient hypoxia as placental blood flow is compromised during contractions in the second stage of labour, and this is usually well tolerated. The fetus that suffers prolonged hypoxia in utero, however, will require active resuscitation at birth.

Transition from the fetal to the normal newborn state requires a range of physiological changes, including aeration of the fluid filled lungs so that gas exchange is transferred from the placental circulation to the lungs of the newborn baby. The normal response to hypoxia of the newborn infant who does not breathe effectively after birth is to become apnoeic ('primary apnoea'); the heart rate is initially normal, but the baby will then become bradycardic as the myocardium becomes hypoxic. The circulation to the brain is preserved initially, but the circulation to the gut, liver, and kidneys is reduced.

If the baby remains hypoxic, gasping respirations will develop. If these efforts fail to aerate the lungs, breathing attempts will fade and the baby will become apnoeic again ('secondary' or 'terminal' apnoea). The baby will then become increasingly hypoxic and acidotic, the heart will fail and the baby will die. This process may take up to 20 minutes in the term newborn. The priority during resuscitation of the newborn is therefore to establish effective aeration of the lungs, so that oxygenated blood is delivered to the heart, cardiac function is restored, and oxygenated blood is delivered to the neural centres in the brain so that respiration is maintained.

Simple ventilation of the lungs is sufficient in the vast majority of cases. If there has been a prolonged hypoxic insult, either in utero or after birth, the baby may also require cardiac compression to deliver oxygenated blood from the lungs to the heart. Some babies who have been severely hypoxic may also require drugs to restore the circulation—the outlook for these babies is poor.

Formal assessment of the newborn is traditionally described using the Apgar score shown in Table 20.1. The score is used to describe the status of the baby at one minute and the response to resuscitation when reassessed at 5 minutes.

Resuscitation of the baby should start immediately if required after delivery, and should not be delayed until the 1-minute score is assessed. A score of 3 is critically low and a score of 7–10 at 5 minutes is normal. A baby who scores less than 7 at 5 minutes should be reassessed every 5 minutes up to 20 minutes. A score of less than 3 at 10, 15 and 20 minutes predicts poor outcome.

20.5.4 Sequence of actions in newborn resuscitation

The sequence of actions required in caring for all newborns includes drying, warmth and assessment, followed by the consideration of **A**irway, **B**reathing, **C**irculation and **D**rugs.

20.5.4.1 *Initial care and assessment*

All newborn babies should be dried, the cord securely clamped, and the baby covered in dry towels to keep warm. Preterm babies (<30 weeks gestational age) should be wrapped in a clean clear plastic bag with the face exposed, and placed under a radiant heater to keep warm. The colour, tone, breathing and heart rate should be assessed rapidly:

- Healthy newborn. Good tone, cries within a few seconds, good heart rate (120–150 beats/min), may be blue initially but turns pink within 90 seconds
- Newborn in need of assistance. Blue at birth, less good tone, may have a slow heart rate (<100 beats/min), may not have established breathing by 90–120 seconds
- Ill newborn. Pale, floppy, not breathing, slow or very slow heart rate.

The heart rate is best assessed using a stethoscope, or if this is not available, by feeling the pulsations in the umbilical cord.

Table 20.1 The Apgar score. The score should be assessed a 1 minute and repeated at 5 minute intervals as indicated

	Score 0	Score 1	Score 2
Colour	Blue or pale	Peripherally blue, centrally pink	Pink
Heart rate	Absent	<100 beats/min	>100 beats/min
Reflex irritability	No response	Grimace	Cry or active withdrawal
Muscle tone	Limp	Some flexion	Active motion
Respiration	Absent	Weak cry: hypoventilation	Good, crying

20.5.4.2 *Airway*

The airway should be opened by placing the baby on his back in the 'neutral' position. Avoid flexion of the neck or overextension, both of which will obstruct the airway.

The airway may be cleared if necessary by gentle suction, but avoid deep suction of the pharynx as this will cause apnoea or bradycardia secondary to vagal reflexes. Do not suction the nose first as this will cause the baby to gasp and inhale mucous and blood from the pharynx. An infant who is floppy may require 'chin lift' or 'jaw thrust' to open the airway. Remember, the priority is to open the airway quickly and for the baby to start breathing, not for extensive suctioning of the airway.

20.5.4.3 *Breathing*

If the baby is not breathing effectively by 90 seconds, give 5 inflation breaths with a self-inflating bag to aerate the lungs. 'Inflation breaths' are defined as sustained breaths of 2–3 seconds up to a pressure of about 30 cm of water pressure.

Reassess the heart rate—if ventilation of the lungs is effective the heart rate should increase and should be maintained above 100 beats/min. Continue low pressure ventilation at a rate of 30–40 breaths/min until the baby starts to breath for himself at a rate of > 30 breaths/min. Intubation may be considered if skilled personnel are available; a size 1 laryngeal mask may be considered as an alternative if tracheal intubation is not available. Remember, bag and mask ventilation is as effective as ventilation via a tracheal tube.

If the heart rate does not increase, reposition the airway and reattempt ventilation – the chest should move with each ventilated breath. Consider oropharyngeal suction, an oropharyngeal airway, or a second pair of hands: one individual to maintain the airway with two hands and the face mask, the second to squeeze the bag.

If the heart rate remains slow (<60 beats/min) or is absent despite adequate ventilation of the lungs, chest compressions may be required.

20.5.4.4 *Chest compression*

If the heart rate fails to respond to effective ventilation, chest compressions may be required. The most effective way to compress the chest in a newborn infant is to place the hands around the chest, with the fingers over the spine at the back and the 2 thumbs pressing on the lower third of the sternum.

The chest should be compressed by approximately one third of the depth of the chest, at a compression rate of approximately 100/min, and a ratio of 3 compressions to one breath.

20.5.4.5 *Drugs*

If the baby has been severely hypoxic, ventilation and compressions may not be adequate to restore the circulation; drugs may be required. However, drugs are not the first line treatment and will be ineffective unless the baby is adequately ventilated (+/– chest compressions if required).

The recommended drugs and doses are described in Table 20.2. They may be delivered via an umbilical venous catheter or a peripheral vein—flush the cannula with 0.9% saline after drugs are given.

If there is a history suggestive of blood loss from the baby, or the baby is shocked with poor peripheral perfusion, a bolus of 10 ml/kg 0.9% saline should be given and may be repeated if required.

Naloxone is not recommended as one of the drugs of resuscitation, but may be given in a dose of 100mcg/kg IM after ventilation and circulation have been established, if the mother has received opioid analgesia in the 4 hours prior to delivery.

Table 20.2 **Drugs used in resuscitation of the newborn**		
Drug (Concentration)	**Dose**	**Comment**
Adrenaline (1:10,000)	10mcg/kg adrenaline (0.1 ml/kg of 1:10,000 solution) If this is not effective, a dose of up to 30mcg/kg may be tried (0.3 ml/kg of 1:10,000 solution)	Adrenaline may be given by IV or via intraosseuous route if the heart rate remains <60 beats/min after adequate ventilation is established The tracheal route is ineffective
Sodium bicarbonate (4.2% i.e. 0.5mmol/ml)	1–2 mmol/kg bicarbonate (2–4 ml/kg of 4.2% solution of bicarbonate)	Bicarbonate should only be given IV once ventilation is secured, ideally after confirming severe metabolic acidosis Higher concentration of bicarbonate solution should not be used as they are too hypertonic
Dextrose (10%)	250mg/kg dextrose (2.5 ml/kg 10% dextrose)	Dextrose should only be given if the blood sugar is low (or if the baby has not responded to adrenaline and bicarbonate) It should not be given routinely during resuscitation.

20.5.5 **Meconium**

Meconium aspiration syndrome is a serious cause of morbidity and mortality in babies with fetal distress. However, many interventions to prevent meconium aspiration have not been shown to be of benefit.

If a baby is born through thick meconium and is unresponsive or is not vigorous at birth, the mouth should be inspected and suctioned to clear the meconium. If there is an individual who is skilled at intubation, the baby may be intubated to clear the larynx and trachea prior to initiating ventilation.

If the baby is born through meconium but is already vigorous, it is not recommended that the baby is intubated to clear the meconium.

It is no longer recommended to suction the nose and mouth of babies to clear meconium when the head is still on the perineum.

20.5.6 **Air versus oxygen**

The use of oxygen or air in newborn resuscitation remains controversial as there are concerns about oxygen toxicity and the development of neonatal encephalopathy.

It has been shown that newborn infants may be resuscitated effectively with either air or 100% oxygen; the most important intervention is to aerate the lungs to allow gas exchange to occur. High concentrations of oxygen should be avoided if possible, particularly in preterm infants.

If the baby fails to improve when resuscitated with air, or if the baby remains cyanosed, then supplementary oxygen should be considered. A baby who has arrested will respond more quickly to resuscitation with 100% oxygen rather than room air.

20.6 **Cessation of resuscitation attempts**

Babies who show any sign of life at birth should be resuscitated unless the gestational age, birth weight or congenital abnormalities render resuscitation attempts futile.

The precise limits for gestational age and weight depend on the local circumstances; a baby of less than 28 weeks gestational age is unlikely to survive in the absence of sophisticated neonatal intensive care. A baby of <23 weeks gestational age or <400 g body weight is unlikely to be viable in any circumstances.

Resuscitation should be stopped if there are no signs of life after 10 minutes of adequate and continuous resuscitation and the baby should be given to the mother to hold if she wishes. If the Apgar score remains less than 3 after 20 minutes the chance of death or severe brain damage is extremely high and it may be justifiable to stop resuscitation efforts.

20.7 **Post resuscitation management**

All infants who have been resuscitated require careful monitoring for at least four hours after delivery. The oxygen saturation should be monitored, particularly where there has been meconium; supplementary oxygen or ventilatory support may be required (CPAP or positive pressure ventilation).

The baby should be kept warm, ideally in skin-to-skin contact with the mother. Overheating should be avoided. The benefits of moderate cooling (34–35°C) for babies who have been severely hypoxic have not been proven.

Blood glucose should be maintained in the normal range; both hyperglycaemia and hypoglycaemia may be detrimental. Newborn infants should be encouraged to breast-feed within the hour; babies who have been severely hypoxic may require supplementary oral or intravenous fluids.

Babies who have been severely hypoxic in utero or after birth may have significant ischaemic damage to the brain, kidneys, liver, or gut, and may have on-going respiratory difficulties; these infants require specialist on-going care.

Index

177

181